Protocols for Gynecologic and Obstetric Health Care

Protocols for Gynecologic and Obstetric Health Care

Mary K. Barger, M.P.H., CNM (Editor)
Assistant Clinical Professor
Department of Community and Family Medicine
University of California, San Diego, School of Medicine

Judith T. Fullerton, Ph.D., CNM
Associate Clinical Professor
Department of Community and Family Medicine
University of California, San Diego School of Medicine
Assistant Dean for Joint Programs at UCSD
University of California, San Francisco, School of Nursing

Vanda R. Lops, M.S.N., CNM
Assistant Clinical Professor
Department of Reproductive Medicine
University of California, San Diego, School of Medicine

Mary Ann Rhode, M.S., CNM
(formerly)
Assistant Clinical Professor
Department of Community and Family Medicine
University of California, San Diego, School of Medicine

W.B. SAUNDERS COMPANY

Harcourt Brace Jovanovich, Inc.

Philadelphia • London • Toronto • Montreal • Sydney • Tokyo

W. B. SAUNDERS COMPANY
Harcourt Brace Jovanovich, Inc.

The Curtis Center
Independence Square West
Philadelphia, PA 19106–3399

Library of Congress Cataloging-in-Publication Data

Protocols for gynecologic and obstetric health care.

　　Includes index.
　　1. Gynecology.　2. Obstetrics.　3. Medical
protocols.　I. Barger, Mary K.　[DNLM: 1. Gynecology—
standards.　2. Obstetrics—standards.　3. Primary
Health Care.　WP 100 P9665]
RG103.P76　1988　　　618.1　　　87–31558
ISBN 0–8089–1897–4

International Standard Book Number　0–8089–1897–4
Printed in the United States of America
10　9　8　7　6　5　4

ACKNOWLEDGMENTS

We want to recognize and thank the nurse-midwives of the University of California, San Diego Nurse-Midwifery Service, past and present, especially Virginia Copeland, CNM, and Patricia Prather, CNM, whose protocols formed the basic outline for this book. It was their hard work in formulating these protocols which encouraged us to write this book so others would have a resource for their practice instead of "starting from scratch."

We would also like to thank Drs. Robert Barmeyer, Ralph Kazer, Thomas Key, Charles Nager, and William Swartz for their invaluable input in reviewing the medical management of this book.

Lastly, we thank Sylvia Johnson and Jan McPheeters for their excellent secretarial assistance in the generation of this manuscript.

CONTENTS

CHAPTER 4
Care of the Menopausal Woman   77

CHAPTER 5
Antepartum Management   87

CHAPTER 6
Intrapartum Management   143

CHAPTER 7
Postpartum Management   171

PREFACE

One goal of health care professionals engaged in the provision of primary care in gynecology and obstetrics is to provide that care in as comprehensive a manner as possible. To do so requires a knowledge base built on expertise developed by both the medical and nursing professions. It is not possible for busy professionals to be proficient in all areas of medical and nursing practice. There is, however, a need for all to be knowledgeable about basic medical and nursing care, teaching and counseling, and psychosocial needs. Basic medical and nursing education programs focus mainly on the content ascribed to their respective professions and usually do not adequately prepare the clinician with essential knowledge from the other discipline.

The purpose of this book, then, is to combine the contributions made to patient care by both the medical and the nursing professions into one concise outline of primary care gynecology and obstetrics.

Because this book is both relatively comprehensive and relatively concise, it should have many uses. It could easily be used as:

1. An educational resource for medical, nurse practitioner, and nurse-midwifery students; physician's assistants; interns; and beginning obstetric/gynecology and family practice residents, all of whom need to function as effectively as possible, while continuing their education.
2. An educational resource for nurses and nurse clinicians requiring a more detailed knowledge of medical management in order to optimize their nursing care.
3. A review for both students and experienced health care professionals.
4. A quick reference for management of situations within the scope of primary care obstetrics and gynecology not commonly encountered by the individual clinician.
5. An orientation outline for new employees in obstetric or gynecologic settings.
6. An example of a very detailed protocol for women's health care assessment and management for those clinicians involved in the development of a protocol for a specific practice setting.

Chapter 1 is an overview of basic physical assessment and the types of services which comprise primary care obstetrics and gynecology. It also includes a summary of selected special situations which may be encountered in a practice. Subsequent chapters provide a more detailed outline of management in the areas of well-woman gynecology, contraception, menopause, antepartum, intrapartum, and postpartum care as appropriate to a variety of birth settings. Each chapter addresses the purpose of the examination or encounter, essential assessment, management, appropriate teaching and counseling, and necessary follow-up or referral. New or controversial assessment techniques or management strategies are referenced so the reader can easily locate further information on the subject.

This book outlines primary care in obstetrics and gynecology. It does not address the management of complex obstetric or gynecologic problems, discussion of high-risk perinatal nursing care, or information such as etiology or pathophysiology. This information is, of course, available in other medical and nursing texts.

While we stress the need to pay attention to a woman's psychosocial needs, it is difficult to summarize psychosocial skills such as empathy and sympathy. We do, however, indicate those situations where a referral to a mental health professional is indicated.

We began writing this book with the intention of helping individuals who need to develop a protocol for a specific practice setting. Later, we realized that the sample protocol we developed had far broader utility than we had anticipated. For those who will use this book to assist them in the development of protocols, the following information may be helpful:

1. A protocol is a written and signed agreement between health care providers. Protocols establish standards and/or limits of practice.
2. Protocols are not a "cookbook." They are a record of an agreement between the providers in the setting, not a substitute for that agreement.
3. Because protocols are a record of a social interchange which has led to an agreement about standards and limits of practice, they can and probably should differ among practice settings. A small private practice with a staff which confers frequently may find a less elaborate record of agreements makes possible more flexible care, while not sacrificing standards. A large practice's protocols may need to be quite detailed in order to avoid misunderstandings and to make orientation of new personnel easier.
4. Personnel should be aware of the legal ramifications of their protocols, and especially, of situations where appropriate care of the patient appears to be at odds with the protocols. We stress that protocols are a mere record of what should be an ongoing, living dialogue performed in the interests of improving patient care.

It is important to remember that medications, diagnostic methods, and therapeutic regimens will change as new research is completed and new technology becomes available. The reader is encouraged to be alert for new developments in medical and nursing practice which may call for alterations in the management outlined herein. Women in need of primary care in obstetrics or gynecology deserve no less than comprehensive, compassionate, and up-to-date management.

Chapter 1

Overview of Essential Health Assessment and Management

Mary Ann Rhode   *Judith T. Fullerton*

This chapter is an overview of the essential assessment and management skills necessary for examining females. Components of a basic physical examination are included as are the requirements for examinations at various ages and for various situations related to reproductive health.

How much to include in a physical examination is always a dilemma. Time is often limited, and a very detailed physical examination may not be appropriate to the presenting problem or situation. However, most women of reproductive age do not seek professional health care unless it is within the context of obstetrical or gynecological care. Health problems unrelated to the reproductive system may be overlooked if a comprehensive examination is not performed. The physical examination outline that follows represents the basics of a comprehensive examination. Although the examination may vary according to the age of the woman, the presenting problem, the purpose of the visit, and the physical setting, each examination should be as comprehensive as possible. Alertness for medical problems unrelated to the reproductive system or laboratory values indicating a need for further investigation, consultation, and referral is essential. This outline presumes the practitioner has basic history-taking and physical assessment skills. More in-depth information on physical assessment techniques may be found in textbooks on physical assessment such as those by Bates,[3] and Malasanos et al.[19]

In the second part of the chapter, variations appropriate to different ages, life cycle events, and special situations are addressed in outline form. Essential components of assessment and management for each type of examination and situation are presented. More detailed discussions of pregnancy, well-woman gynecology, and menopause are provided in subsequent chapters. Further information regarding special situations may be found in the writings cited in the reference list.

1

I. Overview of essential health assessment and management

A. Vital Signs

1. Temperature
2. Blood pressure
3. Pulse rate and regularity
4. Respiration
5. Height and weight (see Tables 1-1 and 1-2 for standard weights for height)

B. General Survey, Skin, and Movement

1. Evaluate general appearance, including symmetry and integrity, body build, and posture.
2. Observe congruence of weight for height.
3. Begin skin inspection with the hands and arms and continue throughout the exam. Observe pattern of hair growth, lesions, and pigmentation.
4. Integrate musculoskeletal evaluation with the exam.
5. Evaluate coordination by observing gait, heel/toe walk, tandem walk, and balance (Romberg).
6. Check for full range of motion of back and for scoliosis and lordosis.

C. Upper Extremities

1. Inspect and palpate hands and nails.
2. Palpate radial and brachial pulses.
3. Palpate epitrochlear nodes for size, consistency, and tenderness.
4. Test range of motion of fingers, wrists, elbows, and shoulders and strength of hands and arms.
5. Check coordination with use of rapid alternating movements and point to point testing.

D. Head and Neck

1. Observe face for symmetry of movement for integrity of the facial (7th) cranial nerve.
2. Palpate skull for symmetry.
3. Inspect scalp and hair.
4. Palpate pre- and post-auricular nodes; occipital, tonsillar, submaxillary and submental nodes; anterior and posterior cervical nodes; and the supraclavicular nodes for size, consistency, and tenderness.
5. Check for tracheal deviation and palpate the thyroid.
6. Palpate or percuss frontal and maxillary sinuses.
7. Palpate temporomandibular joint while patient opens and closes mouth.
8. Palpate temporal and masseter muscles with jaw clenched (5th cranial nerve: trigeminal).

Table 1-1
Table of Desirable Weight for Height*

Height (in.)	Desirable Weight (lbs.)	90% Desirable Weight (lbs.)	135% Desirable Weight (lbs.)
56	101	91	136
57	104	94	140
58	106	95	143
59	109	98	147
60	112	101	151
61	115	104	155
62	119	107	161
63	122	110	165
64	126	113	170
65	130	117	176
66	134	121	181
67	138	124	186
68	142	128	192
69	147	132	198
70	151	136	204

Weight Adjustments for Women 18-24 Years

Age	Subtract Pounds
24	-1
23	-2
22	-3
21	-4
20	-5
19	-6
18	-7

*For women age 25 or over, height without shoes, weight without clothes.

Table 1-2
Mean Weight for Height and Age

Height	Height	Age at last birthday					
(in feet, inches)	(in inches)	12	13	14	15	16	17
4'5" - 4'6¾"	53 - 54.9	65	—	—	—	—	—
4'7" - 4'8¾"	55 - 56.9	84	82	—	—	—	—
4'9" - 4'10¾"	57 - 58.9	88	93	93	106	116	96
4'11" - 5'0 ¾"	59 - 60.9	97	98	106	110	114	110
5'1" - 5'2 ¾	61 - 62.9	107	110	113	114	117	121
5'3" - 5'4 ¾"	63 - 64.9	117	117	120	126	127	127
5'5" - 5'6 ¾"	65 - 66.9	121	128	129	134	136	134
5'7" - 5'8 ¾"	67 - 68.9	140	128	142	144	140	137
5'9" - 5'10 ¾"	69 - 70.9	—	—	135	140	160	145

Maternal and Child Health Branch, California Department of Health Services. (1987). Nutrition During Pregnancy and the Early Postpartum Period. (Draft #3). Sacramento, California: California Department of Health Services (in press). With permission.

9. Test sternocleidomastoid and trapezius muscles against resistance (11th cranial nerve: spinal accessory).
10. Check neck mobility through full range of motion.

E. Ears

1. Test integrity of the acoustic (8th cranial) nerve.
2. Test auditory acuity with whisper test.
3. Test for auditory lateralization (Weber test).
4. Test for air and bone conduction (Rinne test).
5. Palpate and inspect pinnae.
6. Perform otoscopic exam of canals and tympanic membranes.

F. Eyes

1. Test visual acuity (2nd cranial: optic nerve).
2. Inspect external eye.
3. Test visual fields by technique of confrontation.
4. Check extraocular movements in six cardinal positions (cranial nerves 3, 4, and 6: oculomotor, trochlear, and abducens, respectively).
5. Elicit corneal light reflex (Hirschberg's reflex).
6. Check convergence of the eyes during accommodation.

    7. Check pupillary equality and test pupillary reaction to light and accommodation.

    8. Perform fundoscopic examination after eliciting the red reflex.

G. Nose and Oropharynx

1. Inspect external nose.
2. Examine internal nasal structures for deviation, polyps, and exudate.
3. Inspect lips, buccal mucosa, gums and teeth, hard palate, and pharynx. Note moisture, ulcers, nodules, and dentition.
4. Test tongue for strength and symmetry (12th cranial nerve: hypoglossal).
5. Test gag reflex or rise of the soft palate (cranial nerves 9 and 10: glossopharyngeal and vagus nerves, respectively).

H. Lungs and thorax

1. Inspect the skin, contour, and respiratory movements of the anterior and posterior thorax.
2. Palpate for fremitus, tenderness, and symmetry of respiratory excursion.
3. Percuss lung fields bilaterally, and measure diaphragmatic excursion.
4. Auscultate all five lobes, including the apices, for a full inspiration and expiration at each site.

I. Cardiac

1. Inspect and palpate precordium and neck vessels.
2. Auscultate the carotids and valvular areas, with the diaphragm and the bell, with the patient both lying and sitting.
3. Palpate peripheral pulses.
4. Auscultate aortic, pulmonary, right ventricular, and left ventricular areas noting pulsations, thrills, vibrations, and murmurs through all heart sounds of the cardiac cycle.

J. Breasts

1. Instruct client in self-examination while performing the exam.
2. Inspect the breasts with the client in four positions (sitting, arms overhead, hands on hips, and leaning forward) noting size, symmetry, and color.
3. Palpate supra- and subclavicular area noting masses or tenderness.
4. Evaluate the nipples for eversion and erosion by inspection, and evaluate for discharge by gentle expression.
5. Palpate all four quadrants of both breasts and axilla with patient lying down, using radial or transversing techniques. Note size, shape, consistency, tenderness, and nodularity.

K. Abdomen

1. Inspect skin for contour, symmetry, and integrity.

2. Auscultate bowel sounds in all four quadrants.
3. Auscultate over aorta, renal, and femoral arteries.
4. Percuss extent of liver dullness at midclavicular line (MCL) and splenic dullness along the left anterior axillary line (AAL).
5. Palpate for liver edge in right upper quadrant with inspiration.
6. Palpate for tip of spleen.
7. Palpate inguinal area for nodes.

L. Lower extremities

1. Inspect skin and vessels and palpate for temperature, tenderness, and edema.
2. Evaluate femoral, popliteal, dorsalis pedis, and posterior tibial pulses.
3. Test range of motion of ankles, knees, and hips and strength of legs and feet.
4. Check coordination with rapid alternating movement, point-to-point testing, and heel-shin test.

M. Neurologic

1. Evaluate mental status to extent appropriate.
2. Test cranial nerves as part of HEENT exam.
3. Perform sensory testing of all four extremities with light touch and for dull and sharp, vibratory, and position sense; use light touch and test dull and sharp sense on face.
4. Test deep tendon reflexes (biceps, triceps, brachioradialis, patellar, and achilles) and plantar reflex.
5. Integrate motor testing in extremity exams.
6. Integrate and/or test cerebellar coordination at the beginning or the end of the examination.

N. Pelvic

1. Inspect external genitalia for configuration, noting lesions and scars.
2. Palpate Skene's and Bartholin's glands.
3. Perform speculum examination to observe vagina and cervix.
4. Perform bimanual exam to evaluate uterus and adnexa, noting contour, nodularity, position, and size.
5. Perform rectal exam.

II. Essential assessment and management relative to the reproductive system

A. Newborn/infant[1,7,19]

1. Carry out careful examination of genitalia and urethral meatus to rule out ambiguity of sex and abnormalities (such as undescended testicles).

    2. Provide parent education regarding physical characteristics and infant care specific to the female infant.
      a. Breast engorgement
      b. Vaginal skin tags
      c. Withdrawal bleeding
      d. Vaginal discharge
    3. Provide parent education regarding physical characteristics and infant care specific to the male infant.
      a. Breast engorgement
      b. Whether to circumcise
        • Care of the circumcised male
        • Care of the uncircumcised male

B. Child[1,7,19]

    1. Perform physical exam of external genitalia and urethral meatus with reassurance to parent and child of normal findings
    2. Screen for abnormalities.
      a. Vulvitis
      b. Vaginitis or vaginal discharge due to trichomonas, monilia, gonorrhea, pin worms, foreign body in the vagina
      c. Condyloma acuminata and latum
      d. Urethritis
      e. Clitoral hypertrophy
      f. Varicosities, lymphedema, hernia, masses, vaginal adhesions, or pubic lice.
      g. Vulvar hematoma or bruising; document carefully, especially if there is any possibility of sexual molestation, and report to appropriate authorities
    3. Provide opportunity for questions regarding bodily acceptance, sexuality, masturbation, and hygiene.

C. Preadolescent[1,7,19]

    1. Perform physical exam of external genitalia with reassurance to parent and preadolescent of normal findings.
    2. Assess development of secondary sexual characteristics in the manner described by Tanner (Table 1-3).
    3. Screen for abnormalities of the reproductive system.
    4. Educate preadolescent regarding male and female anatomy, physical changes in puberty, and menstruation.
    5. Provide opportunity for questions regarding sexuality and body image.

D. Adolescent[8, 22]

    1. Obtain history in the following areas:
      a. Menstruation
      b. Sexual activity and contraceptive use

  c. Nutritional status and preferences
  d. Drug history, including smoking
  e. Problems or questions identified by the adolescent
2. Perform breast exam and pelvic exam, Pap smear, gonorrhea and/or *Chlamydia* culture, or wet mounts, if indicated.
3. Assess development of secondary sexual characteristics in the manner described by Tanner (Table 1-3).
4. Teach breast self-exam.
5. Teach or review female anatomy, menstruation, and the reproductive cycle.
6. Teach male anatomy and physiology.

Table 1-3
Tanner Staging: Developmental Stages of Secondary Sex Characteristics

Stage	Female Breast Development	Male Genital Development	Male and Female Pubic Hair Development
1	Preadolescent: elevation of papilla only	Preadolescent: testes, scrotum, and penis are about the same size and proportion as in early childhood	Preadolescent: no public hair
2	Breast bud stage: elevation of breast and papilla as small mound; enlargement of areolar diameter	Enlargement of scrotum and testes; skin of scrotum reddens and changes in texture; little or no enlargement of penis	Sparse growth of long, slightly pigmented downy hair, straight or slightly curled, appearing chiefly at the base of the penis or along the labia
3	Further enlargement and elevation of breast and areolar with no separation of their contours	Enlargement of the penis, which occurs at first mainly in length; further growth of testes and scrotum	Hair darker, coarser, and more curled; spreads sparsely over the pubes
4	Projection of the areola and papilla to form a secondary mound above the level of the breast	Increased size of penis with growth in breadth and development of glans; futher enlargement of the testes and scrotum; increased darkening of scrotal skin	Hair adult in type but area covered is still considerably smaller than in the adult; no spread to the medial surface of the thighs
5	Mature stage: projection of papilla only due to recession of the areola to the general contour of the breast	Genitalia adult in size and shape	Adult in quantity and type

Data from Tanner J: Growth at Adolescence. Oxford, England; Blackwell Scientific Press, 1962.

7. Provide opportunity for discussion of the decision to become sexually active, values of parents, peer pressure, self-esteem, the importance and demands of parenting (including the financial and emotional committment) pregnancy, sexually transmitted disease, and substance abuse.
8. Identify and discuss effective methods of contraception and how to obtain them when the decision to become sexually active has been made.
9. Discuss commonly known but ineffective methods of contraception.

E. Interconceptional care

1. History
   a. Family history
   b. Past medical and surgical history
   c. Menstrual history
   d. Obstetrical history
   e. Sexual history
   f. Contraceptive history
   g. Psychosocial history
   h. Personal health habits (e.g., smoking, alcohol, and sexual orientation)
2. Physical examination (age appropriate)
3. Laboratory studies
   a. Complete blood count
   b. Urinalysis
   c. Pap smear
      • Follow American Cancer Society Guidelines
         — First exam at onset of sexual activity or by age 20.
         — Age 20-65: after two negative exams 1 year apart, Pap smear at least every 3 years
      • Some institutions have chosen to continue more frequent monitoring of high risk clients and/or the general population.
   d. Cultures or wet mount for vaginal infections, if indicated
   e. Mammography (see Chapter 2 for American Cancer Society Guidelines)
4. Health education and counseling
   a. Provide contraceptive information, if appropriate
   b. Discuss sexuality and specific areas of concern
   c. Review or teach breast self-exam

F. Pregnancy (see Chapter 10)

G. Perimenopausal, menopausal, postmenopausal gynecological care

1. History
   a. Family history
   b. Past medical and surgical history
   c. Menstrual history
   d. Obstetrical history
   e. Sexual history

      f. Contraceptive history

      g. Psychosocial history

      h. Personal health habits (e.g., smoking, alcohol, and sexual orientation)

   2. Physical examination (see Chapter 4)

   3. Laboratory studies

      a. Complete blood count

      b. Urinalysis

      c. Pap smear yearly

      d. Annual or biannual mammography depending on breast exam

   4. Health education and counseling

      a. Provide education regarding symptoms, causes, and measures for control of discomforts of menopause.

      b. Teach preventive measures for osteoporosis and hip fracture, including diet, exercise, and calcium supplements.

      c. Allow opportunity to discuss changing concepts of sexuality, body image, and femininity.

      d. Provide emotional support as necessary.

      e. Refer to menopause clinics or support groups if desired.

H. Special situations

   1. **Physical abuse** (exclusive of sexual assault)[4,6,10,21]

      a. Be alert for injuries with inappropriate explanations, unusual conditions such as chronic psychosomatic or psychosocial complaints, sexual dysfunction, suicidal behavior, or depression as possible symptoms of physical abuse, past or present

      b. Inquire about the possibility of abusive experiences if there is any suspicion.

      c. Assess woman's psychosocial status, particularly with regard to:
- Self-esteem and confidence
- Motivation to leave violent environment
- Problem-solving abilities
- Financial resources
- Potential support systems

      d. Refer to mental health professional for evaluation and counseling.

      e. If identified, carefully document woman's description of number and intensity of violent incidents and resultant injuries in the medical record. Document if woman's children are subject to violence also, as appropriate. Strongly encourage women to report abuse to appropriate authorities.

      f. Perform physical examination to detect physical injury. Document carefully. Photographs may be helpful; get written consent. Examination by nurse practitioners or physician assistants may not be sufficient in some legal jurisdictions.

      g. Make other appropriate referrals:
- Child welfare

- Medical care
- Legal assistance
- Battered women shelters and support groups

2. **Sexual assault**[14,27]

   a. Examinations done after a reported sexual assault must be done with strict adherence to local procedures, which are usually jointly established by legal and medical authorities. Some jurisdictions may require examination at a specific facility or use of special documents or rape kits. Ignorance of the required procedures or failure to carefully follow them may jeopardize prosecution attempts. Examinations by nurse practitioners or physician assistants may not be acceptable in all legal jurisdictions.

   b. Ensure that all personnel coming in contact with sexual assault victims have the necessary information and compassion to be of assistance.

   c. Examinations for sexual assault will commonly include the following:
      - History
        — Menstrual history
        — Contraceptive history
        — Record of last time of coitus prior to assault
        — Injuries
        — Details of the assault, including the following:
          * Description of assailant(s)
          * Penetration, ejaculation, extragenital acts, use of condom.
          * Time of assault.
          * Location of assault.
          * Any provocation by the victim.
        — Use of drugs or alcohol by the victim prior to the assault
        — Has victim changed clothes, bathed, douched, defecated, or brushed teeth since assault?
      - Physical examination
        — Assess clothing status, presence or absence of hair or stains on clothing, general appearance, and mental status.
        — Examine for genital or extragenital trauma, including hymenal and anal status.
        — Perform pelvic examination with *Unlubricated Speculum.*
          * Note discharge, blood, and lacerations.
          * Obtain vaginal saline samples for sperm and acid phosphatase, Pap smear (with request to comment on presence or absence of sperm), Gram stain, and gonorrhea culture (including rectal and oral samples, if applicable).
          * Perform bimanual exam to determine size of uterus to rule out preexisting pregnancy and presence or absence of pelvic hematomas.
        — Obtain blood for serology, blood alcohol, and/or presence of drugs, if appropriate.

— Obtain combings of pubic hair and clipped samples of victim's hair (especially from areas of matted hair), separately packaged and carefully labeled.
  d. Treatment should include the following:
   • Treat injuries appropriately.
   • Treat prophylactically for sexually transmitted diseases and arrange for appropriate follow-up laboratory studies.
   • Arrange for treatment of emotional trauma of the sexual assault victim, both immediate and long-term.
     — Use rape crisis volunteers whenever possible.
     — Involve specially trained counselors, nurses, or psychiatric social workers as early in the examination process as possible.
     — Arrange for long-term follow-up before victim leaves the health care facility.
     — Refer victim to support groups, if desired.
   • Pregnancy prevention if indicated (see Chapter 3).
  e. Carefully document all findings.
  f. Obtain necessary consent forms for particular procedures such as photographs, special tests, and release of information to relevant authorities.
  g. Establish a chain of evidence form for all people handling evidence (local judicial procedures must be followed).
3. **Lesbian health care**[24,28]
  a. Lesbian women's health care involves all aspects of women's health care.
  b. To meet the health care needs of lesbians and ensure their entry into the health care system, health care professionals must do the following:
   • Be sensitive to a woman's statements, reactions, and body language.
   • Be comfortable in asking questions about sexual activity and sexual orientation.
   • Avoid making assumptions based on the woman's sexual orientation.
     — Address contraceptive needs for the woman who is bisexual.
     — Be alert for alcohol or drug abuse, which may be more prevalent among lesbian women due to societal pressure.
     — Be alert for physical and psychological abuse by the lesbian woman's partner as one would for the heterosexual woman's partner.
     — Be knowledgeable about and alert for sexually transmitted diseases common to lesbian women.
     — Recognize that sexual dysfunction may exist for lesbian women also but that they may be reluctant to verbalize this.
  c. Provide education[24,28] on the following:
   • Health teaching appropriate for all women
   • Physiology of female sexual response
   • Signs and symptoms of sexually transmitted diseases common to les-

bians and ways to prevent their transfer
- Alteration of sexual activity during treatment of sexually transmitted diseases

d. Refer to the following:
- Individual or group counseling relative to identified problems.
- Feminist or lesbian support groups or community centers.
- Mental health facilities as appropriate
- Lesbian mother support groups.

4. **Infertility**[9]

a. Initial contact with woman or couple
- Ensure that staff personnel have adequate education and insight to screen or manage the care of individuals seeking help for infertility.
- Determine if the problem fits the definition of infertility (inability to conceive after a year or more of regular sexual intercourse with no contraception).
  — Couples who have been trying to conceive for less than a year may benefit from information about practices most conducive to conception, including the following:
    * Prompt treatment of any reproductive tract infection
    * Education regarding the menstrual cycle, including awareness of physical changes during the cycle and time of ovulation
    * Intercourse frequency: recommended is every other day, to four times weekly
    * Timing of intercourse near ovulation
    * Avoidance of vaginal lubricant, which may be mildly spermicidal
    * Use of female supine position with thighs flexed and hips slightly elevated unless uterus is very retroverted or retroflexed; maintaining position for 30 minutes after intercourse
    * Refraining from urination or douching for at least 30 minutes after intercourse, especially near the time of ovulation
  — Evaluating couples over 30 years of age earlier than 1 year.
- Avoid fragmentation of care. If clinical setting does not have the equipment, resources, or commitment to adequately manage infertility problems, refer woman or couple elsewhere as soon as possible.
- Encourage participation of both partners.

b. Evaluations for infertility will commonly include some or all of the following:
- History
  — Couple's or woman's description of the problem and previous treatment
  — Gynecologic history
  — Contraceptive history
  — Obstetric history
  — Male genitourinary tract history

— Past medical and surgical history
— Family history
— Exposure to drugs, alcohol, cigarettes, and environmental hazards
— Sexual knowledge, practices, and problems and cultural mores
- Physical examination of both partners (coordination of efforts is essential since the male examination is often done by a urologist in a different setting)
- Laboratory examinations as appropriate to history and physical findings
  — Male partner
    * Semen analysis, including split ejaculate semen analysis
    * Testicular biopsy
    * Urethral calibration
    * Cystourethroscopy
    * Vasography
  — Female partner
    * Hormonal analysis
    * Basal body temperature charting
    * Examination of cervix and cervical mucous at mid-cycle
    * Postcoital test
    * Hysterosalpingography
    * Endometrial biopsy
    * Laparoscopy
- Information about treatment measures, including in-depth instruction regarding treatment or support during specific procedures or the entire course of treatment
- Discussion of and assistance in dealing with such feelings as depression, guilt, grief, or anxiety
- Treatment methods available include the following:
  — Female
    * Induction of ovulation
    * Correction of anomalies
    * Cerclage of incompetent cervix
    * Surgical reconstruction of uterus or fallopian tubes
  — Male
    * Improvement of semen quality by pharmacologic agents
    * Correction of anomalies, e.g.:
      □ Undescended testicles.
      □ Hypospadias
      □ Epispadias
      □ Congenital chordee
      □ Deformities of the penis
      □ Urethral strictures, fistulas, and diverticula
      □ Varicocelectomy
      □ Vasovasotomy or vasoepididymostomy

— Couples
  * Education to improve coital technique
  * Artificial insemination
  * Abstention or use of a condom for a period of time to lower antibody titers of woman with positive results to sperm agglutination tests
  * In vitro fertilization
- Provide appropriate assistance for couples undergoing treatment or for whom treatment has failed.
  — Refer for psychosocial counseling if they are unable to cope with infertility diagnosis.
  — Refer to adoption services.
  — Provide or refer for adoption counseling.
  — Refer to adoption support groups.
  — Refer to infertility support groups.

5. **Unplanned pregnancy**
   a. Obtain history, physical examination, and laboratory studies appropriate to pregnancy and woman's decision regarding desired outcome of pregnancy.
   b. Provide health education and counseling
      - Present available alternatives, including the following:
        — Counseling, if pregnancy is causing undue stress in an existing marriage
        — Marriage, if appropriate, and carrying the pregnancy to term and raising the child
        — Single parenthood
        — Adoption
        — Abortion
      - Offer support for decision and referral to any other appropriate agencies.
   c. Counsel regarding reasons for unplanned pregnancy and offer appropriate contraceptive education for the future.

6. **Losses associated with reproduction**[13,16,18,23,26]
   a. Many types of losses associated with reproduction trigger the same emotions of depression and grief, including spontaneous or therapeutic abortion, stillbirth, neonatal death, birth of a malformed baby, or placement of a baby for adoption.
   b. All types of reproductive loss require some common interventions.
      - Physical care and emotional support are needed during the acute experience.
      - Present information clearly and honestly; repeat it as often as needed by the mother or family.
      - Anticipatory teaching regarding the grief process and informing children or friends is important, including the following:
        — Necessity of grief work to avoid prolonged problems with grief

— Symptoms of grief: fatigue, sleeplessness, preoccupation with the loss, guilt feelings, anger, difficulty accomplishing daily activities
— Encouragement to allow these feelings and manifestations to be expressed
— Acknowledgement of the difficulty and distress involved in grief work

- Ensure the availability of support persons important to the mother throughout the experience
- Discuss contraceptive needs and plans for future pregnancy.
- Refer to public health nursing organizations, social workers, crisis intervention nurses, or pregnancy loss support groups.
- Schedule follow-up visits.
- Telephone mother at 1-2 weeks after discharge to allow for expression of feelings, to monitor progress, and to offer additional assistance.

c. Reproductive loss involving a more advanced pregnancy, a malformed baby, or neonatal death may require additional instructions.
  - Help the mother to make choices about her care.
  - Make arrangements for the parents to see or touch the fetus or infant as often as desired, preferably with supportive personnel present.
  - Describe the infant for parents who may not want to see the infant.
  - Offer appropriate remembrances such as photographs, footprints, infant identification bracelets, crib identification cards, or locks of hair to help establish the reality of the pregnancy.
  - Encourage parents to talk about the experience with others and between themselves.
  - Assist with necessary paperwork, disposal of the body, and arrangements for funeral or memorial service.
  - Refer to organizations or support groups dealing with specific malformations or conditions.
  - Refer for genetic counseling if appropriate for future pregnancies.

7. **Adolescent pregnancy**[5,12,22]
  a. History should include all pertinent history for any pregnant woman with special attention to:
  - Nutritional status and habits
  - Drug history, including smoking
  - Psychosocial assessment including the following
    — Maturity level
    — Coping and problem-solving abilities
    — Family, friend, and school support systems
    — Social environment
    — Present level of education
    — Plans and support for continued education, including education for childbirth
    — Career goals

— Financial support
— Plans for baby care
— Extent of involvement of father of baby
— Mother's perceived education needs regarding pregnancy and baby care

b. Physical exam should include all pertinent physical exam components for any pregnant woman with rigorous screening for the following:
  • Low or excessive weight gain or anemia as a result of adolescent dietary habits
  • Developing signs and symptoms of pregnancy-induced hypertension (more common in adolescents)
  • Signs and symptoms of premature labor (more common in adolescents)

c. Perform laboratory studies (see Chapter 5).

d. Health education and counseling should include the following:
  • Effects of substance abuse and smoking on fetus
  • Sexuality and sex education
  • Developmental changes of adolescence and of pregnancy
  • Peer relationships
  • Nutrition requirements during pregnancy
  • Pregnancy options including the following:
    — Rearing the child as a single or young married parent
    — Parent or relative raising the child
    — Adoption
    — Abortion
  • Support for decision regarding pregnancy option and referral to any other appropriate agencies
  • Comprehensive contraception information to prevent future unwanted pregnancy
  • Importance of consistent prenatal clinic attendance
  • Parenting skills for those choosing to keep their babies, including discussion of infant's psychosocial development,[15] and the following:
    — Recognition of child as a separate, unique individual
    — Importance of verbal and sensory stimulation
    — Need for encouragement of exploration of child's environment
    — Need to allow progressive independence
    — Knowledge of stages of growth and development

e. Refer to adolescent pregnancy support groups, school programs for pregnant adolescents, or adolescent prenatal clinics and teen parent groups.

f. Refer to social services for continued follow-up during and after the pregnancy.

g. Refer to public health nursing service or visiting nurse service for visits during pregnancy and continuing postpartum.

REFERENCES

1. Alexander M, Brown M: Pediatric Physical Diagnosis for Nurses. New York, McGraw Hill, 1974
2. Baldwin K, Goodwin, K: The Papanicolaou smear. J Nurse-Midwifery, 30(6):327-332, 1985
3. Bates B: A Guide to Physical Examination (ed 3). Philadelphia, Lippincott, 1983
4. Blair K: The battered women: Is she a silent victim? Nurse Practitioner, 11(6):38-47, 1986
5. Burst H: Adolescent pregnancies and problems. J Nurse-Midwifery, 24(2):19-24, 1979
6. Carmen E, Rieker P, Mels T: Victims of violence and psychiatric illness. Am J Psychiatry, 141(3):378-383, 1984
7. Chow M, Durand B, Feldman M, et al: Handbook of Pediatric Primary Care (ed 2). New York, Wiley & Sons, 1984
8. Felice M: Adolescence, in Levine M, et al. (eds): Developmental and Behavioral Pediatrics. Philadelphia, Saunders, 1983
9. Fogel I, Woods N: Health Care of Women: A Nursing Perspective. St. Louis, Mosby, 1981
10. Forward S, Buck C: Betrayal of Innocence: Incest and Its Devastation. New York, Penguin, 1979
11. Fritz J, Stull K, Wagner N: A comparison of males and females who were sexually molested as children. J Sex Marital Ther 7(1): 54-59, 1981
12. Furstenberg F, Lincoln R, Menken J: Teenage Sexuality, Pregnancy, and Childbearing. Philadelphia, University of Pennsylvania Press, 1981
13. Gordeuk A: Motherhood and a less than perfect child: a literary review. Matern Child Nurs J 5(2): 57-68, 1976
14. Halbert D, Jones D: Medical management of the sexually assaulted woman. J Reprod Med 20(5):265-274, 1978
15. Howard J, Sater J: Adolescent mothers—Self-perceived health education needs. J Obstet Gynecol Neonatal Nurs 14(5):399-404, 1985
16. Kirkley-Best E, Kellner K: Grief at stillbirth: an annotated bibliography. Birth Family J 8(2):91-99, 1981
17. Koss L: Cytology evaluation of the uterine cervix: factors influencing its accuracy. Pathologist 36:401-407. 1982
18. Kowalski K: Managing perinatal loss. Clin Obstet Gynecol 23(4):1113-1123, 1980
19. Malasanos L, Barkauskas V, Moss M, Stoltenberg-Allen K: Health Assessment. St. Louis, Mosby, 1986
20. Maternal and Child Health Branch, California Department of Health Services. Nutrition During Pregnancy and the Early Postpartum Period. (Draft #3). Sacramento, CA: California Department of Health Services (in press)
21. Meiselman K: Incest: A Psychological Study of Causes and Effects with Treatment Recommendations. San Francisco, Josey-Bass, 1979

22. Neinstein L: Adolescent Health Care. Baltimore, Urban & Schwarzenberg, 1984
23. O'Donahue N: Facilitating the grief process. J Nurse-Midwifery, 24(5):16-18, 1979
24. Olesker E, Walsh L: Childbearing among lesbians: are we meeting their needs? J Nurse-Midwifery, 29(5):322-329, 1984
25. Pickwell S, Novak J: Guidelines of the Physical Examination. Unpublished manuscript, University of California, San Diego, 1985
26. Quirk T: Crisis theory, grief theory and related psychosocial factors: The framework for intervention. J Nurse-Midwifery, 24(5):13-16, 1979
27. Rivlin M: Manual of clinical problems in obstetrics and gynecology. Boston, Little, Brown, 1982
28. Sonstegard L, Kowalski K, Jennings B: Women's Health, Volume I, Ambulatory Care. Orlando, FL, Grune & Stratton, 1982
29. Tanner J: Growth at Adolescence. Oxford, England, Blackwell Scientific Press, 1962

Chapter 2

Well Woman Gynecology

Vanda R. Lops   *Mary K. Barger*

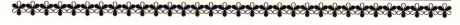

I. Breast exam

A. History
   1. Age: to identify those women at risk for age-associated breast diseases
   2. Presence of masses
   3. Pain
   4. Nipple discharge (spontaneous)
   5. Family history of breast problems
B. Physical assessment (see Chapter 1)
C. Teaching with normal exam
   1. Teach breast self-examination and its importance in early cancer detection. (American Cancer Society recommends monthly breast self-exam after age 20.)[1]
   2. Discuss how to choose proper-fitting and supportive undergarments.
   3. Instruct in breast hygiene.
   4. Encourage breast physical exam according to American Cancer Society Guidelines.
      a. Every 3 years, age 20-40
      b. Every year, over 40
   5. Encourage mammography according to American Cancer Society Guidelines.[1]
      a. Baseline, 35-40
      b. Every 1-2 years, 40-49
      c. Every year, 50 and over
D. **Abnormal exam findings**
   1. Benign fibrocystic breasts
      a. History
         •Patient age may indicate risk status
           —Cysts common in women in 30-50 year age group with cyst formation beginning in mid-20s.
           —Rare in postmenopausal women, since related to ovarian function, especially estrogen production

- Complaints of cyclical breast tenderness, especially premenstrually
b. Physical examination
  - Palpate painful, or nonpainful, often multiple, bilateral breast masses, which are usually round, well-delineated, and mobile.[40]
  - Masses may fluctuate in size and tenderness at different stages of the menstrual cycle.
c. Laboratory studies
  - Mammography and/or ultrasound may be helpful.
  - Biopsy (excisional or needle) may be necessary for definitive diagnosis.
  - Lipid profile helpful in women receiving progesterone, or those at high risk.
  - Refer to physician for endocrine workup if needed.
d. Differential diagnosis
  - Fibroadenoma
  - Carcinoma
  - Papilloma
e. Management and teaching
  - Reassure that findings most probably reflect a normal physiologic state under hormonal influence.[27]
  - Discuss the possiblity of slightly increased risk (two times) for breast cancer even with no other risk factors.[33]
  - Refer to physician for aspiration of cysts and possible biopsy as appropriate, especially if other breast cancer risk factors exist (e.g., mother or sister with breast cancer, nulliparous, previous breast cancer).
  - Prepare the woman for these and other possible diagnostic procedures (e.g., mammography, ultrasound, and endocrine studies).
  - Encourage monthly breast self-exam after menses when tenderness and cysts are at a minimum.
  - Stress importance of the woman's familiarity with her breasts to assist in early detection of potentially malignant masses.
  - Discuss alteration in diet which may ameliorate the condition:
    —Decrease salt intake.
    —Avoid methylxanthines (tea, coffee, colas, and chocolate).[28,36]
    —Decrease fat.
    —Include foods high in vitamin E and vitamin A.[3,12,17,25]
  - Encourage use of padded bra for relief, day and night if necessary.
  - Refer or consult for possible drug therapy, including low-dose oral contraceptives (Loestrin 1/20) or Danazol (100 mg-400 mg, QD) or progesterone.[51]
2. **Nipple discharge**
  a. History
    - Age

- Gravida and parity
- Recent lactation experience or efforts to relactate (e.g., adoptive parent)
- Medication intake, especially oral contraceptives and phenothiazine derivatives
- Symptoms of endocrine system dysfunction (hypothroidism or pituitary adenoma)

b. Physical exam: note type of discharge:
- Serous or serosanguinous
- Multicolored and viscous
- Watery and thin
- Purulent

c. Differential diagnosis
- Galactorrhea
- Intraductal papilloma
- Duct ectasia
- Fibrocystic disease
- Malignancy
- Infection

d. Management and teaching
- Refer for medical consultation.
- Prepare the woman for possible diagnostic tests, including the following[18]:
  —Ultrasound studies (adjunctive modality; may determine cystic versus solid status of mass)
  —Mammography
  —Xeroradiography
  —Cytologic examination of nipple discharge
  —Biopsy
  —Thyroid studies
  —Endocrine evaluation
  —Newer diagnostic aids, still considered experimental (may include graphic stress telethermometry, crystal thermography, diaphanography, and magnetic resonance imaging)
- Prepare the woman for possible therapeutic interventions, including the following:
  —Hormonal therapy
  —Antibiotics
  —Needle aspiration or excisional biopsy where indicated
  —Surgical intervention
- Provide education regarding the following:
  —Need for good breast support, especially during physical activity
  —Importance of proper fitting bra to avoid chafing
  —Medications and diet as prescribed

II. Cervical and vaginal exam

A. History
   1. DES exposure
   2. Age at first intercourse
   3. Multiple sexual partners[34]
   4. History of vaginal infections or pelvic inflammatory disease
   5. Contraceptive history
   6. Obstetric history with attention to manipulative or operative trauma
   7. External lesions
   8. Vaginal discharge: note onset, character, and odor
   9. Vulvar-vaginal irritation, itching, or burning
   10. Dysuria
   11. Dyspareunia
   12. Stress incontinence
B. Physical assessment (see specific diagnostic category for specific assessment requirements)
C. Laboratory studies
   1. Pap smear
   2. Cultures as appropriate (e.g., for gonorrhea, herpes, and/or chlamydia)
   3. Wet mounts
   4. Biopsy as appropriate
D. Teaching with normal exam
   1. Provide reassurance of normal findings.
   2. Offer visualization of anatomy.
   3. Teach Kegel exercises.
   4. Teach pelvic hygiene
      a. Clean perineum from front to back.
      b. Limit douching.
      c. Use tampons properly.
   5. Counsel regarding frequency of physical and pelvic exam.
   6. Provide opportunity for discussion of physiology and sexual functioning.
E. Abnormal exam finding (benign cervical lesions)
   1. History
      a. DES exposure
      b. Reproductive tract anomalies
      c. Exposure to venereal warts
      d. Barrier method contraceptive use and duration of placement during each use
      e. Trauma to cervix (e.g., obstetric trauma, cone biopsies)
   2. Physical examination
      a. Observe for congenital anomalies (double cervix, "cervical atresia," stenosis, congenital absence, congenital shortening, and transverse septum).
      b. Note presence of cervical-vaginal ridging as result of DES exposure (cockscomb cervix).

    c. Observe and describe any polyps (e.g., pedunculated, endocervical, friable).

    d. Describe lacerations, perforations, ulcerations, and growths.

3. Laboratory studies

    a. Pap smear of suspicious lesions or leukoplakia

    b. Cervical cultures as appropriate

Because cytologic reporting of Pap smear results can differ from one institution to another, numerical and descriptive results are given.[32]

I	Normal
II	Atypia due to inflammation (can also list squamous metaplasia), usually no dysplasia
III	Dysplasia, mild, moderate, or severe
IV	Carcinoma in situ (CIS)
V	Invasive cancer

Dysplasia can also be referred to as cervical intraepithelial neoplasia (CIN). This is further classified as follows:

CIN	I	Mild dysplasia
CIN	II	Moderate dysplasia
CIN	III	Severe dysplasia or CIS

---

4. Management and teaching

    a. If so desired, allow the woman to view her entire exam as well as her cervix via a mirror.

    b. Explain findings and their implications for future reproductive health.

    c. Explain implications of DES and need for continued frequent follow-up. Current recommendations regarding the management of DES-exposed women including the following:

      • Initiate pelvic examinations at age 14 or with onset of menses. Exam should include the following:

        —Careful palpation of vagina with special attention to nodularity

        —Careful palpation of cervix with special attention to cervical position and structure

        —Visualization of vagina and cervix for bright red areas or unusual surface contours

      • Cytologic examinations should be conducted.

      • At initial diagnosis of DES, colposcopy and/or biopsy is done. Follow-up colposcopies are done only as indicated.

      • Further follow-up depends on findings.

        —If the exam is normal, yearly follow-up is appropriate.

        —If the exam shows evidence of DES changes, the woman should be referred to physician for 6-month follow-up.

    d. Treat condylomata (see Section IV, J).

     e. If trauma or ulceration is due to barrier method, discuss change in usage pattern, size, or method.

F. Abnormal pap findings (management)
1. Class I: no intervention. Repeat Pap annually or, per American Cancer Society recommendation, every 3 years in low-risk women who have had two consecutive negative smears.
2. Class II. Do wet mount for infectious etiology and provide appropriate treatment, then repeat in 3-4 months, or repeat in 3-4 months, and if still class II, follow above management. If results are persistently class II, colposcopic examination should be done.
3. Class III. Do colposcopic examination.
4. Class IV or V. Refer to physician for follow-up.

III. Uterine exam

A. History
1. Obstetric history
2. Gynecologic history
3. Previous uterine surgery
B. Physical examination
1. Refer to Chapter 1
2. Carefully perform bimanual examination for the following:
   a. Congenital anomalies
   b. Size
   c. Shape
   d. Presence of masses (note consistency, mobility, and tenderness with motion)
   e. Position
   f. Descensus (prolapse)
C. Laboratory study: Pap smear
D. Management and teaching with normal exam
1. Explain size of uterus and position.
2. Discuss implications of position of uterus or degree of descensus on health, possible symptoms, and any necessary interventions.
   a. Teach pelvic rock exercises if retroverted uterus causes low backache.[14]
   b. Fit or refer for pessary if uterine prolapse causes symptoms (usually in older, sexually inactive women).
   c. Refer for surgery as necessary.
3. Teach Kegel exercises to promote adequate support.
E. **Amenorrhea** (Tables 2-1 and 2-2)
1. History
   a. Age
   b. Onset of menses or lack thereof (primary or secondary amenorrhea)
   c. Spotting
   d. Sexual history

Table 2-1
Algorithm for the Evaluation of Patients With Primary Amenorrhea

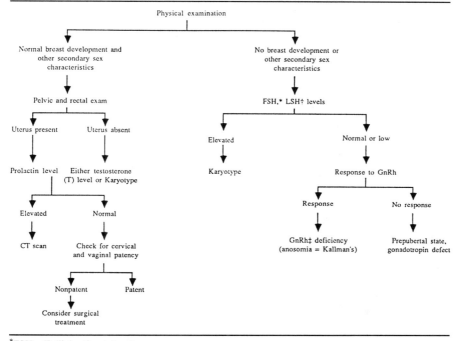

*FSH = Follicle stimulating hormone
†LH = Leutinizing hormone
‡GnRh = gonadotropin releasing hormone

Reprinted with permission from Nichols and Evrard.[36]

    e. Contraceptive history
    f. Exercise patterns (amenorrhea may accompany excessive exercise)
    g. Nutrition patterns (amennorhea may accompany excessive dieting or anorexia)
    h. Obstetric history, especially postpartum hemorrhage and failure to lactate
  2. Physical examination
    a. Observe development of secondary sex characteristics.
    b. Perform careful bimanual exam for congenital anomalies.
  3. Laboratory examination (dependent on history and physical)
    a. Pregnancy test
    b. Vaginal cytology for estrogen effect
    c. Thyroid panel to rule out hypothyroidism
    d. Buccal smear for sex chromatin, if the woman never menstruated

Table 2-2
Algorithm for the Evaluation of Patients With Secondary Amenorrhea

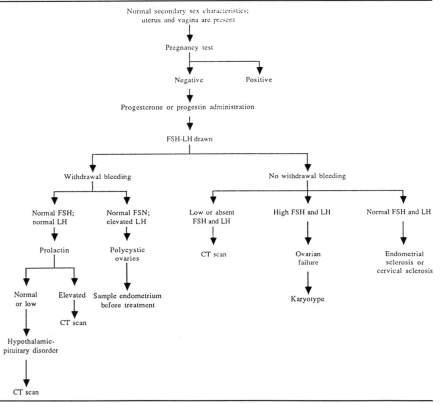

Reprinted with permission from Nichols and Evrard[36]

4. Differential diagnosis
   a. Disorders in the integrity of any one of the four basic compartments necessary for menstruation
      • Uterus
      • Ovaries
      • Anterior pituitary
      • Hypothalamus
   b. Systemic factors
      • Thyroid dysfunction
      • Adrenal dysfunction (Cushing's syndrome)
      • Uncontrolled diabetes
      • Malnutrition
      • Stress and/or depression
   c. Pregnancy

5. Management and teaching
   a. If menstrual pattern has been previously established and pregnancy is
      ruled out, give progesterone challenge: progesterone, 100-200 mg IM,
      or Provera, 10 mg PO QID 5 days. If no response, and the woman is in
      reproductive years, repeat pregnancy test. If negative, refer to physician.
   b. If the woman experiences postpill or postpartum amenorrhea of less
      than 6 months duration, and pregnancy test is negative, reassure her.
   c. Provide or refer for nutritional counseling if malnutrition or eating dis-
      order is present.
   d. Teach stress management techniques as appropriate.
   e. Provide emotional support with explanations of problems and possible
      therapies.[19]
   f. Refer to appropriate support groups.
   g. Refer to physician management according to causal factors.
      • Surgery for anatomic disorders
      • Endocrine workup and/or hormone replacement as indicated
      • Treatment of underlying medical problem

F. **Dysmenorrhea**
   1. History and physical examination
      a. Primary dysmenorrhea
         • Age (patients usually are teens or in early 20s; symptoms begin within
           1 year of menses initiation)
         • Type and location of discomfort
           — Lower abdomen
           — Dull pelvic ache or bearing-down sensation
           — Pain radiating to thighs or lower back
         • Onset and duration of symptoms
           — Symptoms start shortly before or within a few hours of menstrual
             flow.
           — Symptoms usually subside in 12-24 hours but may last 2-3 days
             or throughout entire menses.
           — There is a tendency toward spontaneous alleviation with increas-
             ing age and after childbirth.
         • Present without identifiable gross anomalies
      b. Secondary dysmenorrhea
         • Age (usually older)
         • Location of discomfort
           — Lower abdomen may indicate tubal, uterine, or badder pathology
           — Buttocks and sacral area may indicate vaginal or cervical
             pathology
         • Onset and duration
           — Occurs at different times in menstrual cycle
         • Association with other body functions
           — Defecation
           — Intercourse

— Urination
- Both primary and secondary dysmenorrhea may be accompanied by nausea, vomiting, fatigue, diarrhea, and/or headache
- Additional medical and surgical information
  — Previous or present salpingitis or other pelvic disease (e.g., endometriosis)
  — Previous uterine or surgical surgery
  — Presence of congenital uterine anomaly
  — IUD in place
2. Laboratory studies
  a. Urinalysis and urine culture to rule out urinary tract infection
  b. Cultures as appropriate to rule out pelvic infection
3. Differential diagnosis
  a. Pelvic disease (e.g., endometriosis or PID)
  b. Pelvic anomaly or tumor
  c. Pelvic prolapse
  d. Premenstrual syndrome
  e. Urinary tract dysfunction
  f. Bowel disease
4. Management and teaching
  a. Remove IUD if probable causal factor and observe for improvement
  b. Treat PID if pelvic infection is diagnosed
  c. Treat urinary infection if present
  d. Refer for physician management and further evaluation for the following:
    - Definitive diagnosis of endometriosis
    - Surgical intervention for anomaly, tumor or fibroids, or prolapse
    - Bowel disease
  e. Treat mild symptoms with the following measures:
    - Explain anatomy and physiology of the problem to the woman and reassure her no pathology is present.[52]
    - Encourage balanced diet.
    - Encourage regular, moderate exercise, including lower back and abdominal strengthening exercises.
    - Discuss the use of heat during pain episodes (e.g., heating pad or warm baths).
    - Recommend aspirin for its mild antiprostaglandin effect (650 mg PO TID 1 day before menses begin).
    - If primary dysmenorrhea, advise that the condition will probably improve with time or with childbirth.
  f. Treat moderate to severe symptoms with the following additional measures[37,48]:
    - Order antiprostaglandin medications (e.g., ibuprofen 300,400, or 600 mg PO TID, [10] or naproxen 275-500 mg PO BID).[23]
    - Inform the woman of proper dosage and possible side effects of an-

tiprostaglandins (e.g., mild gastrointestinal upset, thrombocytopenea purpura, or syndrome of nasal polyps, angioedema, and bronchospasm) associated with chronic use. Advise to use with caution with history of asthma.

- Consult with physician if stronger analgesics such as codeine or meperidine (Demerol) are needed.
- Possibly prescribe low-dose (less than 50 μg estrogen) oral contraceptives for 2-3 months (women on birth control pills usually have little dysmennorhea, and relief may continue after discontinuation).[44]
- Teach stress management techniques if stress seems to worsen the dysmenorrhea.

G. **Premenstrual syndrome**
   1. History: elicit presence, severity, cyclicity, and duration of the following symptoms[45]:
      a. Anxiety, irritability, and nervous tension
      b. Edema: 3-5-pound weight increase prior to menses, abdominal bloating, breast congestion
      c. Increased appetite for sweets or other specific foods, especially carbohydrates
      d. Depression, insomnia, fatigue, withdrawal, or thoughts of suicide
      e. Dermatitis with acne
      f. Migraine headache exacerbations
      g. Pelvic discomfort of fullness and congestion
   2. Physical examination
      a. Weigh the woman during luteal phase and after onset of menses to document premenstrual edema.
      b. Examine breasts for tenderness and cystic feeling premenstrually.
      c. Observe skin for premenstrual acne.
      d. Do pelvic exam to rule out other causes of pelvic discomfort.
   3. Laboratory studies
      a. Complete blood count (CBC) and differential: rule out anemia and infection
      b. Chemistry panel: rule out hepatic, renal, and metabolic dysfunction
      c. Glucose tolerance test (if severe hypoglycemic symptoms present)
      d. Thyroid testing (if edema present and persistent)
   4. Management and teaching
      a. Instruct the woman to keep menstrual cycle diary with temperature chart and symptoms.
      b. Counsel the woman regarding the following dietary changes:
         - If hypoglycemic symptoms present, follow hypoglycemic diet: low in sugar, high in protein (50 g/d, limit red meat), and frequent meals to reduce blood sugar fluctuation.
         - If edema symptoms present, restrict sodium premenstrually and increase foods that act as natural diuretics (e.g., strawberries, asparagus, watermelon, and potassium-rich foods).

•If breast congestion occurs, restrict methylxanthines, nicotine, and alcohol.

c. For the following symptoms, supplement diet or eat foods containing the suggested vitamins or minerals
   •Acne: vitamin A and zinc (use only recommended dosages)
   •Depression and irritability: vitamin B_6, 50-200 mg/d

d. Encourage moderate daily exercise, especially for women with anxiety and nervous tension.

e. Teach stress management techniques for symptoms of irritability, withdrawal, or mood swings.

f. Refer for psychological assessment and possible pharmacologic treatment those women with depression or suicidal thoughts.

g. Consult for use of bromocriptine, 2.5 mg PO BID for 10 days prior to menses, to relieve breast congestion.

h. Oral contraceptives may relieve some psychologic symptoms.
   •Prescribe a progesterone-dominant pill for symptoms of anxiety and nervous tension.
   •Prescribe an estrogen-dominant pill for depression, withdrawal, or antisocial behaviors.

i. Provide emotional support or refer to appropriate support groups.

j. Refer to physician management if symptoms worsen or underlying disease is suspected.

H. Dysfunctional uterine bleeding[30,47]

1. History
   a. Age (adolescents and preimenopausal women at higher risk for irregular ovulatory cycles)[35]
   b. Variations in weight (malnutrition, obesity)
   c. Contraceptive use, especially oral contraceptives
   d. Pregnancy exposure
   e. Medical conditions (e.g., hormonal, renal, liver, or blood dyscrasias)
   f. Emotional stress
   g. Strenuous exercise
   h. Onset, regularity, and duration of menses
   i. Onset, amount, and duration of bleeding
   j. Presence of pain or other symptoms associated with bleeding

2. Physical examination
   a. Weigh the woman to document obesity or undernutrition.
   b. Perform general physical exam to rule out medical conditions.
   c. Examine external genitalia for ulcers and lacerations.
   d. Inspect vagina for atrophy, polyps, trauma, lacerations, or carcinoma.
   e. Inspect cervix for ulcerations, polyps, or carcinoma.
   f. Perform uterine exam for motion tenderness, masses, (e.g., fibroids), size, and consistency (rule out pregnancy).

3. Laboratory studies

    a. Complete blood count (CBC) to assess anemia from blood loss and presence of infection

    b. Pregnancy test if pregnancy exposure

    c. Blood chemistry for thyroid, hormonal levels, and clotting factors as appropriate

    d. Pap smear to rule out cancer

    e. Refer to physician as appropriate for the following:
- Colposcopy[42]
- Biopsy of polyps or lesions
- Further endocrine studies
- Endometrial sampling

4. Differential diagnosis

    a. Primary ovarian dysfunction (common in adolescents and peri-menopausal women)

    b. Primary neuroendocrine dysfunction of intrinsic etiology, (e.g., adrenal, thyroid, or hypothalamus) or extrinsic etiology (e.g., drugs, nutritional, or emotional status)

    c. Pregnancy

    d. Atrophic vaginitis

    e. Vaginal abnormalities (tumors, trauma)

    f. Cervical abnormalities (polyps, cancer, endometriosis)

    g. Uterine abnormalities
- Endometritis
- Endometriosis
- Uterine fibroids
- Endometrial hyperplasia
- Endometrial polyps
- Endometrial cancer

    h. Systemic disease

    i. Blood dyscrasias

    j. Oral contraceptive misuse

Nonphysician management primarily includes eliciting and documenting a thorough history and physical. Management will depend on findings and usually will require physician consultation and/or referral.

---

5. Management and teaching: For mild dysfunctional bleeding without systemic symptoms of anemia (and dependent on findings), possible management strategies for a nonphysician provider may include the following:

    a. Counsel the woman regarding appropriate nutrition.

    b. Order iron supplement as appropriate and encourage high iron foods.

    c. Discuss the effects of strenuous exercise on the hormonal system.

    d. Teach stress management techniques or refer for psychosocial counseling as appropriate.

    e. If threatened abortion, give appropriate warnings and encourage bedrest while bleeding.

    f. Treat atrophic vaginitis (see Chapter 4, II, E, 2).

    g. Educate the woman in correct use of contraceptives.

    h. Teach the woman how to maintain a basal body temperature chart and record symptoms during the cycle.

    i. Refer or consult with physician after obtaining information.

I. Pelvic inflammatory disease (PID)

  1. History

    a. Recent medical-surgical history (high-risk women include those with recent pelvic surgery, recent delivery and recent abortion)

    b. Previous PID

    c. Multiple sexual partners

    d. Contraceptive use, especially IUD in place

    e. Last menstrual period (at increased risk day, 5-10 of menstrual cycle)

    f. Onset, location, type, and severity of pain (usually lower abdominal pain radiating to back and possibly the legs)

    g. Systemic symptoms (e.g., fever, chills, nausea, and malaise)

  2. Physical examination

    a. Take vital signs including temperature.

    b. Palpate abdomen for distention, rebound tenderness, and guarding and auscultate for hypoactive bowel sounds.

    c. Examine Skene's glands for inflammation and discharge.

    d. Visualize cervix and vagina for purulent discharge.

    e. Palpate cervix, uterus, and adnexae for motion tenderness (unusual or exquisite), pain, and masses.

  3. Laboratory studies

    a. Obtain CBC with differential (will demonstrate leukocytosis with left shift).

    b. Obtain erythrocyte sedimentation rate (ESR) (may be elevated) or C-reactive protein.

    c. Perform Gram stain of Skene's or cervical exudate (to identify gram negative diplococci).

    d. Culture cervical exudate for gonorrhea

    e. Obtain endocervical swab for *chlamydia* test.

    f. Refer to physician for the following:

      • Culdocentesis: fluid may contain WBCs with or without gonococci or other organisms

      • Ultrasound, to visualize pelvic or adnexal masses, fluid-filled tubes, or fluid in cul-de-sac

      • Abdominal x-ray to demonstrate ileus

  4. Differential diagnosis

    a. Appendicitis

    b. Ectopic pregnancy

    c. Ruptured corpus luteum cyst

    d. Diverticulitis

    e. Septic abortion

    f. Torsion of an adnexal mass

    g. Degeneration of a leiomyoma

    h. Endometritis

    i. Endometriosis

    j. Urinary tract infection (UTI)

    k. Ulcerative colitis

5. Management and teaching

    a. Refer the woman for hospitalization for any of the following:

      • Pelvic abscess is suspected.

      • Temperature is greater than 102.2°F with rebound or abdominal guarding in upper abdomen.

      • She is pregnant.

      • She fails to respond to outpatient treatment in 48-72 hours or is unable to comply with outpatient treatment.[41]

      • She is a prepubertal child or adolescent (controversial if sexual abuse is suspected).

      • Diagnosis is uncertain.

      • There is a surgical emergency (e.g., appendicitis or ectopic pregnancy is suspected).

    b. Centers for Disease Control recommended treatment schedules are as follows[6]:

      • Amoxicillin 3 g PO, or ampicillin 3-5 g PO, or ceftriaxone 250 mg IM, with probenecid, 1 g PO or

      • Aqueous procaine penicillin G, 4.8 million units IM (at two sites), with probenecid, 1 g PO

      Either regimen can be followed with either of the following:

      • Doxycycline, 100 mg PO BID for 10-14 days, or

      • Tetracycline, 500 mg PO QID for 10-14 days

    c. Make sure that the woman understands how to take medicine and potential food interactions.

    d. If IUD in place, consult with physician (removal is usual).

    e. If IUD has been removed, discuss alternative methods of contraception.

    f. The woman must return in 2-3 days after initiation of medication to evaluate progress.

    g. Counsel the woman regarding signs and symptoms of a worsening condition and to contact provider if they occur.

    h. Encourage rest, especially abstinence from sexual activity, until cured.

    i. Discuss use of heat to lower abdomen and over-the-counter analgesics for pain relief.

    j. Refer sexual partner for evaluation and treatment.

    k. Discuss use of condoms to prevent future infections.

    l. Provide support and reassurance.

   m. Schedule the woman to return 7-14 days after completion of therapy
      for evaluation and possible follow-up cultures.
J. Chronic pelvic pain

*This entity may be one of the most challenging to diagnosis. The essential respon-
sibility of the nonphysician care provider is that of data collection followed by
referral or consultation with the physician for therapy regimen.*

   1. History[30,36]
      a. Age
      b. Obstetric experience (especially recent pregnancy)
      c. Pelvic surgery (potential for adhesion formation)
      d. Any recent surgery, especially if complicated by infection
      e. Last menstrual period
      f. Ongoing medical conditions or medications
      g. Onset, duration, character, and location of pain (e.g., lower abdomen,
         vagina, pelvis)
      h. Factors associated with pain (e.g., menses, sex, exercise, rest)
   2. Physical examination
      a. Take vital signs to document infection parameters.
      b. Observe gait of woman for signs of clutching abdomen or "doubling
         up."
      c. Perform "jar test" by having woman stand on toes and drop suddenly to
         her heels. Severe discomfort confirms peritoneal irritation, usually with
         acute rather than chronic pain. [36]
      d. Palpate abdomen for masses and pain and auscultate hypoactive bowel
         sounds (severe peritoneal irritation).
      e. Perform speculum exam of vagina and cervix for discharge, bleeding,
         lesions, masses, IUD string.
      f. Perform bimanual exam to assess uterus and adnexae for size, shape,
         masses, and tenderness.
   3. Laboratory studies
      a. CBC for anemia and infection
      b. Urinalysis and possible urine culture
      c. Pregnancy test as appropriate
      d. Serology test for syphilis
      e. Cervical and vaginal cultures as indicated
      f. Refer to physician for the following:
         • Culdocentesis if PID or ectopic pregnancy suspected
         • Ultrasound for pelvic masses, PID, or pregnancy
   4. Differential diagnosis
      a. Endometriosis
      b. Peritoneal adhesions
      c. PID, acute or chronic
      d. Pelvic relaxation
      e. Bone disease (degenerative)

  f. Chronic urinary tract infection
  g. Hernia
  h. Gastroenteritis, intestinal tumors, or bowel obstruction
  i. Psychogenic
5. Management and teaching
  a. Discuss physical and laboratory findings with the woman.
  b. Treat those conditions within nonphysician provider management.
  c. Teach and encourage daily Kegel exercises if pelvic relaxation a causative factor.
  d. Refer to physician management and outline probable diagnostic and therapeutic regimens as appropriate for the woman.

K. **Endometriosis**
1. History
  a. Dysmenorrhea (lower abdominal pain that increases premenstrually or during menses)
  b. Dyspareunia
  c. Infertility
  d. Abnormal uterine bleeding
  e. Painful defecation
2. Physical examination
  a. Palpate for presence of fixed, retroverted uterus.
  b. Palpate adnexa for thickening, nodularity, or irregular cysts on an ovary.
  c. Palpate for "frozen pelvis" (uterus or adnexae immobile).
3. Laboratory examination
  a. Ultrasound
  b. Laparoscopy
  c. Biopsy of observable lesions
4. Differential diagnosis
  a. Premenstrual syndrome
  b. Adenomyosis
  c. Leiomyomata
  d. Chronic salpingitis
5. Management and teaching
  a. Order ibuprofen or naproxen (doses should be individualized) for pain relief.
  b. Start the woman on continuous oral contraceptives (pseudopregnancy may decrease stimulation and size of endometrial implants).
  c. Alternative therapy: prescribe danazol 400-800 mg PO QD (pseudomenopause may decrease size and stimulation of endometrial implants).
  d. Discuss nature of disease entity and management.
  e. Prepare the woman for further evaluation (e.g., laparoscopy)
  f. Ascertain wishes regarding future pregnancy for counseling if radical surgery (removal of uterus and ovaries) is to be considered.

L. **Toxic shock syndrome (TSS)**
  1. History[7]
     a. Age (more prevalent in younger women)
     b. Regularity and amount of menstrual flow
     c. Tampon use during menstruation
     d. Recent pelvic surgery, including previous tubal ligation
     e. Vaginitis within the last year[24]
     f. Type of contraceptive method used (use of oral contraceptive pills [OCPs] may be protective)[24]
     g. Previous episode of TSS
     h. Onset or presence of fever, rash, gastrointestinal symptoms, muscular myalgias
  2. Physical examination[8]
     a. Take temperature: greater than 38.9°C or 102°F is indicative of TSS.
     b. Monitor blood pressure for hypotension or orthostatic changes.
     c. Observe skin for diffuse macular rash.
     d. Observe palms and soles for desquammation, which usually occurs 1-2 weeks after onset of TSS.
     e. Palpate abdomen for masses or tenderness.
     f. Examine musculoskeletal system for myalgias.
     g. Assess central nervous system for altered consciousness without focal signs.
  3. Laboratory studies[8]
     a. Platelets (< 100,000 suggestive)
     b. Urinalysis for WBCs
     c. Renal function tests (BUN or creatinine two times normal)
     d. Liver function tests (SGPT, SGOT, and bilirubin may be twice normal level)
     e. Cultures of blood, throat, and CSF as appropriate to document presence of *Staphylococcus aureus* and to rule out diseases under differential diagnosis[49]
  4. Differential diagnosis
     a. Kawasaki's disease (characteristically no hypotension, renal failure, or thrombocytopenia present)
     b. Scarlet fever (presents with sore throat, petechiae on soft palate, and strawberry tongue)
     c. Rocky Mountain spotted fever (usually no hypotension, rash appears gradually)
     d. Leptospirosis (culture or serologic evidence confirms this diagnosis)
     e. Rubeola (characteristic Koplik's spots on mucous membranes of mouth)
  5. Management and teaching
     a. Refer immediately for physician managment and hospital admission if TSS is suspected.
     b. For the woman who has recovered from TSS:

- Encourage her to avoid use of tampons.
- Teach proper hygiene.
- Advise that highest risk of recurrence is within next three menses.

   c. Prevention measures for TSS include the following[53]:
- Mechanical rather than manual insertion of tampons
- Frequent tampon changes during menses
- Use of oral contraceptives (may be protective)
- Treatment for suspected vaginitis

M. **Pelvic relaxation syndrome**
   1. History
      a. Obstetric experience (e.g., traumatic delivery, large infants)
      b. Pelvic surgery, especially hysterectomy and oophorectomy
      c. Onset of menopause
      d. Onset and duration of any of the following symptoms:
- Sensation of vaginal fullness or pressure ("falling out")
- Stress incontinence, urinary frequency, or feeling of incomplete bladder emptying
- Difficult elimination of feces
- Lower abdominal pulling or backache

      e. Presence of chronic cough or chronic straining
      f. Other medical conditions (e.g., diabetes)
   2. Physical examination
      a. Observe for obesity.
      b. Observe perineum for bulging or mass at the introitus.
      c. Observe for leaking of urine with full bladder after coughing or bearing down.
      d. Perform pelvic examination to assess the following:
- General tone
- Integrity of anterior and posterior vaginal walls
- Changes in vaginal walls with coughing or bearing down

      e. Perform rectovaginal exam to assess the following:
- Bulging or reducible thickness of upper rectovaginal septum (enterocele)
- Thin-walled rectovaginal septum (rectocele)

   3. Laboratory studies (dependent on diagnosis)
      a. Cath urine for residual volume after voiding and to rule out infection (cystocele or urethrocele)
      b. Cystoscopy (cystocele or urethrocele)
      c. Barium enema (enterocele or rectocele)
   4. Differential diagnosis
      a. Cystocele
      b. Urethrocele
      c. Rectocele
      d. Enterocele
      e. Uterine prolapse

     f. Tumor of bladder or urethra, rectum, or cervix

5. Management and teaching
   a. Prevent pelvic relaxation by instructing woman prenatally and postpartally to do Kegel exercises regularly.
   b. Encourage weight loss in obese women.
   c. Provide estrogen therapy to menopausal women to help maintain pelvic tone.
   d. Correct or avoid chronic cough, constipation, and traumatic deliveries.
   e. If cystocele is present, do the following:
      • Instruct the younger woman to do 100-200 Kegel exercises daily for 6-12 months.
      • Make sure the woman is completely emptying her bladder by reducing cystocele into vagina prior to voiding or by voiding again several minutes after first voiding.
      • Treat any chronic urinary infection.
      • Refer for pessary for temporary relief of symptoms if symptoms persist after above measures.
      • Refer for surgery as appropriate.
   f. If rectocele is present, do the following:
      • Ensure adequate fluids and fiber in diet to avoid constipation.
      • Instruct the woman to apply pressure on posterior vaginal wall to aid in defecation.
      • Refer for pessary as temporary measure as symptoms warrant.
      • Refer for surgery as appropriate.
   g. If enterocele is present, do the following:
      • Refer for pessary and/or surgery as warranted by symptoms.
   h. If uterine prolapse is present, do the following:
      • Refer for pessary and/or surgery as warranted by symptoms.

IV. Sexually transmitted diseases (STDs)

A. **Bacterial vaginosis** (*Gardnerella vaginalis, Hemophilus vaginalis*, nonspecific vaginitis, *Corynebacterium vaginalis*)
   1. History[16]
      a. Presence of malodorous vaginal discharge
      b. Possible mild vulvar irritation
   2. Physical examination[15]
      a. Note presence of typically frothy, grayish malodorous discharge.
      b. Vaginal mucosa may or may not be inflamed.
      c. Cervix may occasionally exhibit small punctate hemorrhages (similar to *Trichomonas*).
   3. Laboratory studies[2]
      a. Vaginal pH is 4.7-6.0.
      b. "Clue cells" (epithelial cells with a stipled or granulated appearance) are present in saline wet mount under x 40 microscopic power.

    c. Positive "sniff test" elicited: when KOH is mixed with discharge it causes a fishy odor.

    d. Gram stain reveals fine gram-negative bacilli with rounded ends in short chains (school of fish) or granular conified cells. Few polymorphonuclear leukocytes or lactobacilli are seen.

4. Differential diagnosis
    a. Other vaginal infections
    b. Other STDs
    c. Cervicitis
    d. Uterine infection
    e. Foreign body in posterior fornix such as a tampon or diaphragm.

5. Management and teaching
    a. Systemic treatment consists of prescribing one of the following regimens[20,22,29]:
- Metronidazole, 500 mg PO BID x 7 days[6]
- Metronidazole, 250 mg PO TID x 7 days
- Ampicillin or amoxicillin, 500 mg PO QID x 7 days (may mask presence of gonorrhea or syphillis, therefore, rule those out prior to treatment)
- Tetracycline, 500 mg PO QID x 7 days (contraindicated in pregnancy and lactating women due to possible retardation of fetal skeletal development and permanent discoloration of the teeth)
- Cephalexin 500 mg PO QID x 7 days

    b. Local treatment may alleviate symptoms but may not cure disease.[46]
- Consider anti-*Monilia* medication prophylactically if antibiotic used.
- Betadine douche may be used once or twice a day to alleviate malodorous discharge.
- Encourage cleansing of irritated vulva with water and vinegar solution two or three times daily.

    c. Treat partner or refer partner for treatment in resistant or recurrent cases.
    d. Explain the nature of the infection and its treatment.
    e. Stress good personal hygiene.
    f. Advise avoidance of sexual intercourse during treatment or use of a condom until completion of treatment.
    g. Stress disinfection of diaphragm or cervical cap if appropriate.

B. *Chlamydia*
1. History
    a. Recent exposure to infected sexual partner (e.g., male partner has urethritis
    b. Sexual history including multiple partners
    c. Presence of grayish or mucoid nonspecific vaginal discharge (symptoms usually mild and the woman may be asymptomatic)
    d. Urinary symptoms as dysuria and frequency.
    e. Vulvar soreness

  f. Presence of PID symptoms
2. Physical examination
  a. Assess for PID (see Section V, E).
  b. Observe cervix for mucopurulent or grayish mucoid discharge.
  c. Observe cervix for friability or signs and symptoms of inflammation (e.g., redness and edema).
3. Laboratory studies
  a. Ascertain vaginal pH (will be >5).
  b. Perform wet mount for numerous polymorphonuclear leukocytes and to rule out *Monilia*, trichomoniasis, and/or bacterial vaginosis.
  c. Culture cervix for gonorrhea and *Chlamydia*, or
  d. Obtain enzyme linked immunoassay (Chlamydiazine) or fluorescein-labeled monoclonal antibody test (Microtrak) (highly specific).
4. Differential diagnosis
  a. Other vaginal infections
  b. Other STDs
  c. Cervicitis from other causes (trauma, chemical, etc.)
5. Management and teaching[4]
  a. Treat the woman with one of the following therapies[6]:
   • Tetracycline HCl, 500 mg PO QID x 7 days, or
   • Doxycycline, 100 mg PO BID x 7 days, or
   • Erythromycin (base or sterate), 500 mg PO QID x 7 days
  b. Treat pregnant women as follows:
   • Women at high risk should be cultured.
   • Prescribe erythromycin, base 500 mg PO QID x 7 days, or erythromycin ethylsuccinate, 800 mg PO QID x 7 days. If nauseated, give one half of daily dose of erythromycin (e.g., 250 mg) PO QID x 14 days.
  c. Advise the woman of mode of transmission, via sexual contact.
  d. Refer all sexual contacts for evaluation and treatment.
  e. Stress need to complete entire course of treatment.
  f. Advise the woman to avoid sexual activity until cured or to use a condom.
  g. Return for test-of-cure 4-7 days posttreatment (may omit if finances and lab resources are limited since cure rates are more than 95 percent). [6]
  h. If pregnant, preterm labor incidence is slightly increased; therefore, discuss symptoms and formulate management plan accordingly.
  i. Answer all questions the woman may have.
C. *Gonorrhea neisseria*
1. History
  a. Exposure to an infected partner
  b. Previous infection or pelvic inflammatory disease
  c. Dysuria, abdominal or pelvic pain, or vaginal or urethral discharge
  d. Skin lesions or pustulant vesicles anywhere on body
  e. Migratory tenosynovitis with purulent synovial effusion

2. Physical examination
    a. Examine lesions if present.
    b. Evaluate joint inflammation if present.
    c. Palpate lower abdomen for tenderness, pain, or masses.
    d. Perform vaginal exam for the following:
        • Presence of discharge from Skene's and/or Bartholin glands
        • Discharge from endocervix
        • Cervical motion tenderness elicited on bimanual exam
        • Evaluation of uterus and adnexa for inflammation and/or masses
3. Laboratory studies
    a. Obtain Gram stain (95 percent useful in males and 40-60 percent useful in females, with an overall 5 percent false-negative rate).
    b. Obtain cultures from appropriate sites (pharynx, endocervix, urethra, and rectum).
    c. Order laboratory tests for concurrent STD (e.g., VDRL).
    d. Refer for synovial fluid culture if indicated.
4. Differential diagnosis
    a. Cystitis
    b. Vaginitis or cervicitis due to other organism
    c. Local versus disseminated gonococcal infection
5. Management and teaching for uncomplicated anogenital GC infection
    a. Prescribe one of the following regimens (single-dose therapies are preferred)[6]:
        • Ampicillin, 3.5 g PO, or amoxicillin, 3.0 g PO, with probenecid, 1 g PO
        • Ceftriaxone, 250 mg IM
        • Aqueous procaine penicillin G (APPG), 4.8 million units IM in two sites, with probenecid 1 g PO
        • Tetracycline, 1 g PO, then 500 mg PO QID x 7 days
        • Erythromycin, 500 mg PO QID x 7 days (for patients allergic to penicillin [PCN])
        • Spectinomycin, 2.0 g IM: use for PCN-resistant organisms only (second drug of choice for PCN-allergic persons)
    b. Any of the above regimens should be followed by one of the following to cover coexistent chlamydial infections (occurs in 45 percent of cases):
        • Tetracycline, HCl 500 mg PO QID x 7 days, or
        • Doxycycline, 100 mg PO BID x 7 days, or
        • Erythromycin (base of sterate) 500 mg PO QID x 7 days
    c. Discuss importance of treatment of all recent sexual partners.
    d. Discuss course and transmission of disease in women. (The woman may be asymptomatic but should PID develop, she may be at high risk for infertility, pain, ectopics, and recurrences.)
    e. Encourage sexual abstinence or use of condom until cured.
    f. Discuss safe sex practices, including the use of condoms.

g. Schedule for follow-up culture for test-of-cure in 7-14 days.

h. Consult or refer to physician if salpingitis (disseminated GC) is diagnosed. Possible drug regimens include the following:
- Aqueous crystalline penicillin G, 10 million units IV daily (minimum 3 days) until improved, followed by amoxicillin or ampicillin, 500 mg PO QID x 7 days
- Ampicillin, 3.5 g PO, or amoxicillin, 3 g PO, with probenecid 1 g PO, followed by Ampicillin or amoxicillin, 500 mg PO QID x 7 days
- Cefoxitin, 1 g IV QID for at least 7 days
- Cefotaxime, 500 mg IV QID x 7 days
- Ceftriaxone, 1 g IV QD x 7 days
- For penicillin- or cephalosporin-allergic patients: tetracycline, 500 mg QID x 7 days, or doxycycline, 100 mg BID x 7 days.

D. **Herpes genitalis** (HSV-II)
  1. History
     a. Previous herpes infection
     b. Fever, headache, and/or malaise (primary infection)
     c. Presence of vesicular lesions, especially with burning or mild parasthesia
     d. Dysuria
     e. Presence of tender, swollen lymph nodes (primary infection)
     f. Sexual partner with HSV-II diagnosis or lesion on penis
  2. Physical exmaination
     a. Palpate inguinal nodes.
     b. Note signs of viremia.
     c. Observe labia, perineum, vagina, and cervix for vesicles or shallow, painful ulcers (may be single or multiple).
  3. Laboratory studies
     a. Obtain cells on a dry slide for a Tzanck smear; presence of giant cells is indicative of herpes.
     b. Culture lesions for herpes virus (Hanks media).
     c. In an asymptomatic pregnant woman, culture entire exocervix and vagina, and perform vulvar sampling of areas where previous lesions have occurred.[5]
     d. Obtain serologic studies at primary episode, then repeat in 7-10 days (a fourfold rise indicates primary infection). [5]
  4. Differential diagnoses: syphillis and abnormal Pap
  5. Management
     a. Ascertain if primary or recurrent infection; primary infection may last 2-6 weeks.
     b. Prescribe acyclovir cream 5%, topical application every 3 hours, 6 times a day for 7 days for primary herpes. Can be used in recurrent episodes to decrease intensity and duration of lesions, but is most helpful in primary occurrence.
     c. Prescribe acyclovir tablets orally as follows:

- Initial outbreak: recommended dose is 200 mg PO every 4 hours while awake for a total of five tablets daily for 7-10 days (initiated within 6 days of outbreak of lesion).
- Intermittent recurrent outbreaks: 200 mg PO QID while awake for total of five tablets daily for 5 days. Therapy should be initiated at earliest sign of recurrence. *Note:* Safety of acyclovir in pregnancy is not fully established and use is not recommended.
- Suppressive therapy for chronic recurrent disease is 200 mg PO TID for up to 6 months. Some clients may require up to 200 mg PO five times daily for up to 6 months.
  d. Prescribe lidocaine ointment 5% applied topically to lesions to decrease pain.
5. Teaching
  a. Counsel that no cure is available and there may be recurrent episodes; however, these are usually of shorter duration.
  b. Discuss associating factors that may trigger recurrence, including fever, menses, and emotional stress. If client can identify triggering factors for herself, she can try to avoid them.
  c. Discuss symptomatic relief measures during episode.
    - Void while pouring warm or lukewarm water over perineum or in bathtub with warm water.
    - Take over-the-counter analgesics for pain relief.
    - Keep lesions clean and dry. Alcohol, camphor, and providone-iodine (Betadine) have been used with varying success for drying of vesicles.
  d. Advise the woman to be cautious about other therapies that purport to cure lesions.
  e. Inform the woman she may infect partner from first signs of burning or itching until lesions have completely dried.
  f. Encourage the woman to have yearly Pap smear.
  g. Advise the woman that if she becomes pregnant, it is important to tell health care provider of her history.
  h. Provide psychological or emotional support to the woman. Refer for professional care if indicated.
  i. Refer to herpes support groups if available.
E. **Human immunodeficiency virus (HIV)**
  1. History and physical examination
    a. The following high-risk populations should be offered screening[13]:
      - IV drug users and partners
      - Prostitutes
      - Spouses and partners of HIV-positive people or people with AIDS or AIDS-related complex (ARC)
      - Clients with medical conditions requiring frequent blood transfusions and/or blood products
    b. Elicit and/or assess for presence of the following:
      - Night sweats

- Fever
- Anorexia
- Extreme fatigue
- Unexplained weight loss
- Lymph node enlargement

2. Laboratory studies: obtain blood for HIV antibody screening
3. Management and teaching
   a. Explain that there is no known cure.
   b. If HIV screen is positive, notify the woman and set up a plan of management for consultation and referral with her.
   c. Practitioners should familiarize themselves with legal statutes regarding patient rights of confidentiality in the case of a positive screen.
   d. Counsel individuals at risk regarding behaviors to reduce that risk.
      - IV drug users should avoid contaminated needles.
      - Teach prevention through safe sex practices, e.g., use of condoms.
      - Advise women to avoid sexual contact with persons known to have AIDS or at high risk to have AIDS.
   e. Educate the woman regarding HIV symptom complex; if HIV-positive woman is pregnant, advise on availability of interruption-of-pregnancy services.
   f. Provide emotional support measures and refer to support groups as appropriate.
   g. Reaffirm confidentiality of laboratory results.

F. **Moniliasis (occasionally a STD)**
   1. History
      a. Complaints of vulvar pruritus and vaginal discharge in relation to menstrual cycle (premenstrual exacerbations often occur due to increase in vaginal glycogen)
      b. Dysuria
      c. Dyspareunia
      d. Use of oral contraceptives
      e. Diabetes or signs and symptoms of diabetes
      f. Antibiotic use
   2. Physical examination
      a. Perform speculum examination for variable amounts of thick, white, curd-like or flocculent discharge.
      b. Examine vagina and vulva for erythema (may be absent).
      c. Examine vulva and inner thighs for cutaneous lesions, small, reddish macules, and vesicopustules. Excoriation is common due to intense puritus.
   3. Laboratory studies
      a. Wet mount with vaginal discharge diluted with 10% KOH for microscopic examination; *Candida* species appear as oval budding cells and pseudomycelia
      b. Dipstick urine for glucose

    c. Urine or vaginal cultures as appropriate (growth will occur in 2-3 days)
4. Differential diagnosis
    a. Other vaginal infections (5-10 percent of *Trichomonas* infections have concurrent candida)
    b. Chemical vulvovaginitis or cervicitis
    c. Atrophic vaginitis
    d. Leukoplakia
    e. Neurodermatitis (allergic reaction)
    f. Allergic reactions
5. Management
    a. Prescribe one of the following:
- Butoconazole nitrate 2% vaginal cream: one applicator nightly for three nights
- Clotrimazole 500-mg single-dose vaginal tablet or 1% vaginal cream (one applicator) or 100-mg vaginal tablets nightly for 7 nights (longer therapy recommended for recurrent infection or pregnant women)
- Miconazole 200-mg vaginal suppositories nightly for three nights or 2% vaginal cream (one applicator) every night for 7 nights
- Nystatin, 100,000-unit vaginal suppository once daily for 7-14 days

    b. Alternative therapies include the following:
- Cultured plain yogurt: one applicator in vagina twice daily (acidophilus in yogurt restores lactobacilli in vagina)
- Boric acid, 600 mg in size 0 gelatin capsules, one tablet every day for 7 days, then two times a week for 3 weeks, if recurrent infection[50]

    c. Refer to physician:
- If there is a superimposed bacterial or viral infection
- If chronic dermatitis of skin on vulva or thighs develops

    d. Pregnant women near term should be treated since the neonate may develop skin or mucous membrane infection and, rarely, systemic candidiasis.
6. Teaching
    a. Discuss the nature, predisposing factors, and treatment of the infection.
    b. Suggest warm sitz baths to relieve discomfort from vulvar involvement.
    c. Complete entire course of medication even if symptoms disappear.
    d. Continue medication through the menses if necessary.
    e. Keep area dry and exposed to air as much as possible.
    f. Practice good personal hygiene, including frequent bathing and wiping from front to back after bowel movement.
    g. Wear loose fitting cotton underwear since it is more porous and retains less moisture and heat than nylon.
    h. Avoid pantyhose and tight-fitting slacks or jeans.
    i. Women who experience chronic or recurrent infection may use medication at bedtime 7-10 days prior to menses. (Increased vaginal glycogen at that time supports reinfection.)

    j. Avoid using feminine hygiene sprays, bath oils, and strong soaps on vulva or in vagina; they may cause allergy or irritation.

    k. Reduce sugar and refined carbohydrate intake if excessive.

    l. Screen for diabetes if infections are recurrent or nonresponsive to therapy.

    m. Be sure sexual partner is free from infection to prevent reinfection.

    n. Avoid intercourse during treatment or use a condom.

    o. Take precautions against reinfection from fomites, bath towels, soiled clothing, diaphragm, etc.

    p. Oral contraceptive or chronic antibiotic users with recurrent or chronic infections may need to consider an alternate birth control method and treatment methods.

G. Pediculosis pubis

  1. History

    a. Known exposure

    b. Presence of itching in pubic area

  2. Physical examination

    a. Examine pubic hair for egg casing (nits) on hair shafts.

    b. Note presence of erythematous macules, papules, or secondary excoriation of genital area.

    c. Check inguinal lymph nodes for enlargement.

  3. Laboratory studies using a magnifying class, identify a small (1 cm) squat body with claws, giving organism a crab-like appearance

  4. Differential diagnosis any other cause of pubic itching

    a. Dermatitis

    b. Vaginitis

    c. Scabies

  5. Management[21]

    a. Prescribe one of the following therapies:

      • Lindane 1% lotion or cream. Apply to infested area and wash off in 8 hours. Medication may be reapplied at weekly intervals.

      • Lindane (Kwell) shampoo. Apply to affected and surrounding hairy areas for 4 minutes, then wash off and dry. Use a fine-tooth comb to remove remaining nit shells.

        — Reapplication may be repeated in 24 hours but no more than twice in a week.

        — Contraindicated in pregnancy.

      • Pyrethrins and piperonyl butoxide can be used.

        — Apply to affected and surrounding hairy areas for 10 minutes, then wash off.

        — This is the preferred treatment in pregnancy.

    b. Re-treat in 7 days if lice or eggs are observed.

  6. Teaching[21]

    a. Stress importance of following directions for use of medications correctly.

b. Complete entire treatment.

c. Disinfect clothing and bedding by washing in hot water with bleach if possible, or dry clean.

d. Avoid sexual or close physical contact until treatment is completed.

e. Evaluate partners or other family members for need of treatment.

f. Return in 1 week if not cured or if infection recurs.

H. **Syphilis**

1. History

a. Previous or recent exposure to infected sexual partner

b. Multiple sexual partners

c. Prostitution

d. Previous positive serum serology

e. Presence of genital lesions

f. Complaints of rash, skin lesions, mucous patches, or condylomata lata (secondary syphilis)

g. Complaint of systemic symptoms, including malaise, headache, and fever (secondary syphilis)

2. Physical examination

a. Examine oral and genital area, including vagina and cervix, for lesions, including red papule, ulcer, or painless, indurated chancre (primary syphilis).

b. Observe skin, especially genital area, for rash, skin lesions (may look like scabies), mucous patches, and condylomata lata (secondary syphilis).

c. Palpate lymph nodes for enlargement (primary or secondary syphilis).

3. Laboratory studies

a. Using darkfield microscopy, examine exudate from primary and secondary lesions for *T. pallidum*. (Important since serum tests do not become positive until 4 weeks after appearance of chancre.)

b. Order a rapid plasma regimen (RPR) or venereal disease research laboratory (VDRL) screening test.

   • These are nonspecific antibody tests for syphilis. (False-positive reactions have been identified in women with vaccinia infectious, mononucleosis, certain viral infections, and long-standing collagen disease such as lupus and arthritis.)

   • RPR and VDRL may change from positive to negative 1 year after adequate treatment.

c. If screening test is positive, order a treponomal-specific test:

   • Fluorescent trepenoma antibody absorption (FTA-ABS)

   • Trepenoma immobilization test (TPI)

   • *T. pallidum* hemagglutination antibody (TPHA)

d. If tertiary syphillis is suspected, refer for spinal tap for evaluation of cerebrospinal fluid (rule out neurosyphilitis).

4. Differential diagnosis

a. Yaws

    b. Pinta: chronic, dyschromic dermatosis caused by *Trepenoma carateum*

    c. Bejel: nonvenereal syphilis occuring in the Middle East

  5. Management

    a. Diagnose type of syphilis.

- Primary: patient has typical lesion(s) and a newly positive serology test there is a fourfold increase over previous titer; and syphilis exposure has occurred within the previous 90 days.
- Secondary: patient presents with rash or lesions and a strongly positive serology test.
- Latent: patient is asymptomatic but has serological evidence of untreated syphilis.
- Tertiary: disease is of more than 3 years duration with symptoms involving cardiovascular, neurological, and dermatological systems.

    b. Refer all cases of tertiary syphilis to physician.

    c. Treat primary, secondary or early syphilis of less than 1 year duration. Treatments are listed in preferred order.

- Benzathine penicillin G 2.4 million units IM or
- Tetracycline HCl, 500 mg PO QID for 15 days (for penicillin-allergic patients) or
- Erythromycin (sterate, ethyl succinate, or base), 500 mg PO QID x 5 days (treatment of choice only for penicillin-allergic, tetracycline-intolerant, or pregnant patients)

    d. Treat syphilis of indeterminate length or more than 1 year's duration with the following:

- Benzathine penicillin G, 7.2 million units total, 2.4 million units IM once a week x 3 weeks or
- Tetracycline, 500 mg PO QID x 30 days (for penicillin-allergic patients) or
- Erythromycin, 500 mg PO QID x 30 days (treatment of choice only for penicillin-allergic, tetracycline-intolerant, or pregnant patients)

  6. Teaching

    a. Stress importance of completion of therapy.

    b. Identify sexual contacts and arrange for treatment.

    c. Advise woman to refrain from intercourse or to use condoms until follow-up tests of self and partner are negative.

    d. Discuss implications of infection on pregnancy and delivery as appropriate (spontaneous abortions, neonatal conjunctivitis).

    e. Teach signs and symptoms of medication side effects and how to take oral medication.

    f. Stress importance of follow-up serologies at 3, 6, 12, and 24 months after therapy.

I. **Trichomoniasis**

  1. History[31,43]

    a. Profuse vaginal discharge with severe itching

    b. Dyspareunia, dysuria, and urinary frequency

    c. Postcoital spotting, menorrhagia, or dysmenorrhea (rare) due to increased pelvic vascularity wrought by extensive trichomoniasis

2. Physical examination

    a. Examine external genitalia for redness, swelling, and tenderness.

    b. Note presence of profuse, frothy gray or greenish malodorous vaginal discharge.

    c. Examine cervix or vagina for inflammation or punctate submucosal hemorrhages (strawberry spots).

3. Laboratory studies

    a. Wet mount of exudate in saline solution to identify flagellated trichomonads

    b. Though rarely utilized, vaginal/cervical culture for trichomonads may be helpful

4. Differential diagnosis

    a. Other vaginal infections

    b. Other STDs

    c. Uterine infection

    d. Cervicitis

    e. Urinary tract infection

5. Management and teaching

    a. Order metronidazole 2 g PO (single-dose treatment) or 250 mg PO TID x 7 days.[26]

      • Avoid alcohol during and 3 days following therapy since it may cause nausea, vomiting, and headache.

      • Gastrointestinal symptoms are common even if alcohol is avoided.

      • Patient may experience sharp, metallic taste.

      • Use with caution in pregnancy.

    b. An alternative therapy for the pregnant woman is clotrimazole cream, one applicator every night x 7 days (50% cure rate)[38]. If metronidazole must be prescribed in pregnancy, attempt to limit use to last two trimesters and dosage schedule over 7 days can be utilized.[9]

    c. Use topical intravaginal preparations for temporary relief of symptoms but note that long-term cure rates (by culture at 3 months) are less than 30% since infection remains in extravaginal sites, including periurethral glands and endocervix.

      • Betadine douche, 2 tablespoons to 1 quart of lukewarm water, use once daily.

      • Topical steroid cream for severe vulvar irritation; use sparingly three times a day until relief is achieved.

    d. Carefully explain to the woman that most cases are sexually transmitted and partner, though asymptomatic, should be treated.

    e. Reassure that if properly treated and eradicated, the organism will not damage the genitourinary tract.

f. Offer women, particularly adolescents, opportunity to see the viable trichomonad under the microscope as an additional incentive to take medications properly.

g. Instruct the woman to return promptly for reexamination if symptoms have not completely abated within 7 days or if symptoms of vulvovaginitis or pelvic pain recur at any time thereafter.

h. Women who demonstrate an abnormal Pap smear of the cervix repeated 6 weeks or more after metronidazole treatment for trichomoniasis should receive appropriate referral for colposcopy.

i. Advise women to avoid use of tampons during treatment since they may absorb some of the vaginal medication.

j. A strongly acid douche (2 tablespoons of vinegar to 1 quart of warm water) after intercourse with an infected male may be helpful.

k. Refrain from intercourse during treatment, or use a condom.

l. Refer to physician for the following:
   • Superimposed bacterial infection
   • Persistent class II or III Pap smear after treatment of infection
   • Unusual pelvic tenderness

J. Venereal warts (*Condylomata acuminata*)

1. History
   a. Age of onset of sexual activity (correlates with young age)
   b. Multiple sexual partners
   c. Presence of vaginal discharge, usually with foul odor

2. Physical examination
   a. Examine vulva, perineum, anus, and vagina and cervix for single or multiple soft, fleshy, possibly pedunculated growths varying in size from a pinhead to large masses covering entire vulva.

3. Laboratory studies
   a. Order wet mount to rule out vaginitis.
   b. Obtain Pap smear if cervical lesions are present.
   c. Biopsy atypical lesions to rule out carcinoma.
   d. Refer for colposcopy if flat warts are a possible diagnosis (possibly linked to cervical dysplasia).[11]
   e. Obtain serology test for syphilis to rule out *Condylomata lata*.

4. Differential diagnosis
   a. Carcinoma
   b. *Condylomata lata*

5. Management and teaching
   a. Apply podophyllin 10% in tincture of benzoin topically to growths (limit application to growths on external vulvar area) and wash off in 1-4 hours (or sooner if pain occurs). Repeat 1 to 2 times weekly up to four applications.
   • Protect normal tissue by applying petroleum jelly to area surrounding treatment area and to opposite side.

•If warts persist after four weekly treatments, refer for alternative therapy.

•Do not use in pregnancy or with cervical, urethral, oral, or anorectal warts.

b. Refer to physician for one of these alternative therapies as appropriate:

•Cryosurgery, cauterization, or surgical incision (preferred for pregnancy)

•Trichloroacetic acid topically applied

•5-Fluorouracil topically applied for extensive flat condylomata of cervix and vagina

•Carbon dioxide laser surgery (most effective method for vaginal flat condylomata and pedunculated lesions of vulva); apply cold tea compresses for analgesia following laser therapy

c. Refer to physician any pregnant woman whose warts enlarge to point of obstructing the birth canal.

d. Encourage the woman to return weekly or biweekly for treatment until lesions have resolved.

e. Instruct the woman that her partner should be examined for warts.

f. Advise the woman to abstain from sex or to use condom during therapy.

REFERENCES

1. American Cancer Society: Recommendations for the early detection of cancer in asymptomatic people. CA 35(4):XX,1986

2. Amsel R, Totten P, Spiegel C, et al: Nonspecific vaginitis; Diagnostic criteria and microbial and epidemiologic associations. Am J Med 74(1):14-22, 1983

3. Band P, Deschamps M, Falardeau M, et al: Treatment of benign breast disease with vitamin A. Prev Med 13(5):549-554, 1984

4. Bourcier K, Siedler A: *Chlamydia* and *condylomata* acuminata: An update for the nurse practitioner. JOGN Nurse 16:17-21, 1987

5. Brown Z, Berry S, Vontuer L, et al: Genital herpes simplex infections complicating pregnancy: Natural history and peripartum management. Reprod Med 31 5 (suppl): 420-425, 1986

6. Center for Disease Control: STD treatment guidelines. MMWR 34(45):745-1065, 1985

7. Chesney P, Bergdoll M, Davis J, et al: The disease spectrum, epidemiology, and etiology of toxic-shock syndrome. Annu Rev Microbiol 38:315-338, 1984

8. Chow A, Wong C, MacFarlane A, et al: Toxic shock syndrome: Clinical and laboratory findings in 30 patients. Can Med Assoc J 130(4):425-430, 1984

9. Creasy R, Resnik R: Maternal-Fetal Medicine. Philadelphia, Saunders, 1984

10. Dawood M: Ibuprofen and dysmenorrhea. Am J Med 77(1A):87-94, 1984

11. Deitch K, Smith J: Cervical dysplasia and condylomata acuminata in young women. JOGN Nurse 12:155-158, 1983

12. Ernster V, Goodson W, Hunt T, et al: Vitamin E and benign breast "disease": A double-blind, randomized clinical trial. Surgery 97(4):490-494, 1985
13. Finkbeiner A, Hancock E, Schneider S: AIDS. Johns Hopkins Magazine 38:15-27, 1986
14. Finneson B: Low Back Pain. Philadelphia, Lippincott, 1980
15. Fleury F: The clinical signs and symptoms of *Gardnerella*-associated vaginosis. Scand J Infect Dis 49:71-72, 1983
16. Goei S, Wells J: *Corynebacterium vaginale* in nonpurulent vaginitis. Med J Aust 1(9):470-472, 1983
17. Goldstein P: The effect of vitamin E on mammary dysplasia: A double blind study. Obstet Gynecol 65(1):104-106, 1985
18. Green F, Hicks C, Eddy V, et al: Mammography, sonomammography, and diaphanography: A prospective, comparative study with histologic correlation. Am Surg 51(1):58-60, 1985
19. Greenberg R, Fisher S: Menstrual discomfort, psychological defenses, and feminine identifiction. J Pers Assess 48(6):643-648, 1984
20. Hagstrom B, Lindstedt J: Comparison of two different regimens of metronidazole in the treatment of non-specific vaginitis. Scand J Infect Dis 40:95-96, 1983
21. Hatcher R, Guest F, Stewart F, et al: Contraceptive Technology 1986-1987 (ed 13). New York, Irvington Press, 1986
22. Hovik P: Nonspecific vaginitis in an outpatient clinic. Comparison of three dosage regimens of metronidazole. Scand J InfecT Dis 40(suppl):107-110, 1983
23. Kauppila A, Ronnberg L: Naproxen sodium in dysmennorhea secondary to endometriosis. Obstet Gynecol 65(3):379-383, 1985
24. Lane S, Poole C, Dreyer N, et al: Toxic shock syndrome, contraceptive methods, and vaginitis. Am J Obstet Gynecol 154(5):989-991, 1986
25. London R, Sundaram G, Murphy L, et al: The effect of vitamin E on mammary dysplasia: A double-blind study. Obstet Gynecol 65(1):104-106, 1985
26. Lossick J: Single-dose metronidazole treatment for vaginal trichomoniasis. Obstet Gynecol 56(4):508-510, 1980
27. Love S, Gelman R, Silen W: Fibrocystic "disease" of the breast—A non-disease? N Engl J Med 307(16):1010-1014, 1982
28. Lubin R, Rone E, Waxy Y, et al: A case-control study of caffeine and methylxanthines in benign breast disease. JAMA 253(16):2388-2392, 1985
29. Malouf M, Fortier M, Morin G, et al: Treatment of *Hemophilus vaginalis vaginitis*. Obstet Gynecol 57(6):711-714, 1981
30. Martin P: Handbook of Office Gynecology. Orlando, FL, Grune & Stratton, 1985
31. Mason P: Trichomoniasis: New ideas on an old disease. S Afr Med J 58(21):857-859, 1980
32. Morrow P, Townsend D: Synopsis of Gynecologic Oncology. New York, Wiley and Sons, 1981

33. Myhre E: Is fibrocystic breast disease a pre-malignant state? Acta Obstet Gynecol Scand 123:189-191, 1984
34. Newton W, Keith L: Role of sexual behavior in the development of pelvic inflammatory disease. J Reprod Med 30(2):82-88, 1985
35. Ngu A, Quinn M: Dysfunctional uterine bleeding in women over 40 years of age. Aust NZ J Obstet Gynaecol 24(1):30-33, 1984
36. Nichols D, Evrard J: Ambulatory Gynecology. Philadelphia, Harper & Row, 1985
37. Owen P: Prostaglandin synthetase inhibitors in the treatment of primary dysmenorrhea. Am J Obstet Gynecol 148(1):96-103, 1984
38. Rein M: Current therapy of vulvovaginitis. Sex Trans Dis 8(4 suppl): 316-320, 1981
39. Richardson J, Cigtay O, Grant E, et al: Imaging of the breast. Med Clin North Am 68(6):1481-1514, 1984
40. Saltzstein S: Potential limits of physical examination and breast self-examination in detecting small cancers of the breast. Cancer 54(7):1443-1446, 1984
41. Salvio K, Apuzzio J: New antibiotics in the treatment of pelvic infections. JOGN Nurse 13(5): 308-311, 1984
42. Sheppard B: The pathology of dysfunctional uterine bleeding. Clin Obstet Gynaecol 11(1):227-236, 1984
43. Spence M, Hollander D, Smith J, et al: The clinical and laboratory diagnosis of *Trichomonas vaginalis* infection. Sex Transm Dis 7(4):168-171, 1980
44. Starks G: Therapeutic uses of contraceptive steroids. J Fam Prac 19(3):315-321, 1984
45. Steege J, Stout A, Rupp S: Relationships among premenstrual symptoms and menstrual cycle characteristics. Obstet Gynecol 65(3):398-402, 1985
46. Steinmetz K: *Gardnerella vaginalis vaginitis:* A guide to identification and management for the practitioner. J. Nurse-Midwifery 31(2):87-92, 1986
47. Strickler R: Dysfunctional uterine bleeding in ovulatory women. Postgrad Med 77(1):235, 1985
48. Stromberg P, Akerlund M, Forsling M, et al: Vasopressin and prostaglandins in premenstrual pain and primary dysmenorrhea. Acta Obstet Gynecol Scand 63(6):533-538, 1984
49. Todd J: Staphylococcal toxin syndromes. Annu Rev Med 36:337-347, 1985
50. VanSlyke K, Michel V, Rein M: Treatment of vulvovaginal candidiasis with boric acid powder. Am J Obstet Gynecol 141(2):145-148, 1981
51. Vorherr H: Fibrocystic breast disease: Pathophysiology, pathomorphology, clinical picture, and management. Am J Obstet Gynecol 154(1):161-179, 1986
52. Wilson M: Menstrual disorders, premenstrual syndrome, dysmenorrhea, amenorrhea. JOGN Nursing, 13(suppl 2): 11s-19s, 1984
53. Witzig D, Ostwald S: Knowledge of toxic shock syndrome among adolescent females: A need for education. J School Health 55(1):17-20, 1985

Chapter 3

Contraception

Mary K. Barger

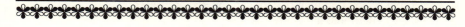

I. Purpose of visits

A. Evaluate woman's knowledge of contraception and ability to act on her knowledge.

B. Evaluate woman's attitudes about sexuality and how this is influenced by culture and religion.

C. Evaluate woman's attitudes about pregnancy, abortion, and contraception.

D. Obtain history of sexual and contraceptive practice, including successes and failures.

E. Assist woman to choose a contraceptive method that meets her particular needs.

F. Provide adequate teaching so that the woman may safely maximize the effectiveness of the chosen method.

II. Steroidal contraceptives: combined oral and phasic pills

A. History
   1. Absolute contraindications include the following[7]
      a. Known or suspected cancer of the breast or history thereof
      b. Known or suspected estrogen-dependent neoplasia or history thereof
      c. Thrombophlebitis, thromboembolic disease, or history thereof
      d. Cerebrovascular accident or disease
      e. Undiagnosed uterine bleeding
      f. Known or suspected pregnancy
      g. Benign or malignant liver tumor (or history)
      h. Known impaired liver function at present time
   2. Relative contraindications include the following[6,12]:
      a. Hypertension
      b. Migraine headaches
      c. Diabetes or prediabetes
      d. Active gallbladder disease
      e. Active phase mononucleosis
      f. Sickle cell (SS) disease or sickle C (SC) disease

g. Age of 45 or older

h. Age of 35-40 and heavy smoking (15 cigarettes or more a day)

i. Lactation: estrogen decreases milk supply

B. Physical assessment

   1. Baseline weight

   2. Blood pressure

   3. Pelvic exam with Pap smear

C. Laboratory studies (prior to institution of therapy)

   1. Two-hour postprandial screening test if prediabetic or having a strong family history (normal <130 mg/100 mL)

   2. Lipid screen if at high risk for cardiovascular disease[10]

D. Management of initial therapy

   1. Initiate on 35 μg of estrogen or less to prevent estrogen side effects

     a. Combined pills

- These provide the same combination of estrogen and progestin each day for 21 days.
- They are packaged in 21-day or 28-day cycles (the last week is a placebo).
- Ortho-Novum 1/35 or Norinyl 1/35 are widely used for initiation.

     b. Multiphasic pills

- These provide varying doses of progestin with a constant level of estrogen during the cycle for 21 days.
- The incidence of breakthrough bleeding is similar to that of combined pills.[17]
- Advantages are as follows:
  — Less progestin (other oral contraceptive pills [OCPs] can give lower progestin throughout the cycle)
  — Fewer metabolic effects secondary to less progestin
- Disadvantages are as follows:
  — Confusion of patient and clinician secondary to the multicolor coding of pills
  — Difficult for clinician to assess side effects and correct the problem when two or three different pills are used

   2. Special considerations

     a. Hirsute women or women with acne: initiate on a low androgenic potency pill (Ovcon-35, Modicon, or Brevicon).

     b. Borderline serum lipid values or strong family history of cardiovascular disease: initiate on a low-progestin-activity pill (Ovcon-35, Modicon, or Brevicon or multiphasic pills).

     c. Women with the following conditions may be treated with 80-100 mcg estrogen pills (for contraception no woman should be started at this dose):

- Ovarian cysts
- Dysfunctional uterine bleeding
- Severe acne (Enovid)

- Endometriosis
d. Women taking medications that accelerate estrogen breakdown, i.e., Dilantin or Rifampin: initiate on 50 μg estrogen pills.
3. Have woman sign informed consent regarding risks and benefits of oral contraceptives (see Section G).
4. Provide woman with 3-6 cycles supply of oral contraceptives.
5. Woman will need to return prior to finishing her last cycle.
E. Management of continued therapy
1. Return after initial 3-6 cycles to monitor weight, blood pressure, symptoms, and compliance.
2. Give seven cycles of pills if no problems and blood pressure normal.
3. If a problem, refer to management of complications.
4. Schedule return for annual exam.
F. Management of complications and side effects
1. Hypertension (140/90 on three separate visits):
   a. Change to progestin-only pill.
   b. Evaluate BP over next 3-6 months.
   c. If hypertension continues, discontinue all hormones.
   d. Inform woman that hypertension due to hormones is usually reversible in 1-3 months after discontinuation.
   e. Encourage woman to make lifestyle changes that may be contributing to hypertension, including stopping smoking, decreasing weight, and increasing exercise.
2. Mild headache
   a. Utilize headache evaluation form to differentiate vascular from nonvascular types (several forms are available).[7]
   b. If migraine type headache, use progestin-only pill or nonhormonal contraceptive.
   c. If clearly associated with fluid retention, change to lower estrogenic active pill.
3. Nausea
   a. Obtain history regarding duration, severity of nausea, and relationship to OCP intake and other possible etiologies.
   b. Rule out pregnancy by inquiring about other symptoms or performing appropriate tests as indicated.
   c. Tell woman that nausea usually decreases after the first few cycles.
   d. If vomiting occurs within 1 hour of intake, tell woman to take another pill from a separate pack.
   e. Encourage woman to take pill with evening meal or at bedtime.
   f. If nausea persists, change to a less estrogenic pill.
4. Acne
   a. Determine onset and duration of symptoms to rule out other causes, including allergy, stress, and polycystic ovarian disease.
   b. Change to a low androgenic potent pill or change to a higher estrogenic active pill.

    c. If no improvement or worsening of symptoms, woman may need to discontinue oral contraceptives.

    d. Encourage the use of drying agents, such as benzoyl peroxide, or refer for more extensive treatment.

5. Chloasma

    a. May worsen with sun exposure; encourage consistent use of SPF 15 sunscreen.

    b. Change to a pill with less estrogenic activity.

6. Depression, mood change, and/or fatigue

    a. Obtain history regarding past depressive episodes, timing in relation to pill use, severity, and presence of causative factors (e.g., loss of job or change in a relationship).

    b. Administer a self-rating depression inventory (Beck) to confirm depression versus fatigue and decreased libido.

    c. Assure adequate vitamin B (especially B_6: 25 mg daily) to rule out depression caused by decreased pyridoxine.

    d. If fatigue is the primary complaint, change to lower progestin-dose pill.

    e. If irritability occurs on pill-free days and there is no cyclic edema, increase estrogenic potency.

    f. If irritability occurs with cyclic edema, decrease estrogenic potency.

    g. If depression is present and clearly related to pill use, discontinue pills for three to six cycles and observe for improvement.

    h. If depression is severe or preceded pill use, refer woman to an appropriate mental health professional.

7. Weight gain

    a. Obtain history to determine pattern of weight gain, affected body areas, changes in appetite, and pregnancy symptoms.

    b. If cyclic gain, use low estrogenic potent pill.

    c. If chronic or gradual gain, use low androgenic potent pill or progestin-only pill.

    d. Provide dietary counseling to reduce caloric intake and encourage exercise to maintain appropriate weight.

8. Spotting or breakthrough bleeding[15]

    a. Obtain history on the following:

      • Dosage, duration, and consistency of pill use

      • Duration, amount, and timing of spotting

      • Past or present history of gynecologic problems, including pelvic pain, dyspareunia, and vaginal discharge

      • Symptoms of pregnancy

      • Use of drugs interfering with OCPs, including phenobarbital and rifampin

    b. Perform appropriate exams to rule out pathology based on history or symptoms.

    c. Correct any problems or misunderstandings in timing and consistency of pill use.

d. Assure woman is receiving adequate dose.
- If vomiting and diarrhea occur within 1 hour of taking pill, take another pill.
- Increase dose in presence of drugs that interfere with OCPs.
e. If symptoms occur during first four cycles of pill use, and woman is taking pills correctly, reassure woman that problem will probably resolve by the fourth cycle.
f. If after initial four cycles symptoms persist, change to a higher progestin-active pill no matter where the bleeding occurs in the cycle.[3]
g. If bleeding continues, do one of the following:
- Change to a higher estrogen-active pill,[3] or
- Supplement OCPs with additional exogenous estrogen (2.5 mg conjugated estrogen or 20 µg ethinyl estradiol), daily for 7 days when bleeding is present, irrespective of where the woman is in the pill cycle.[15]
h. If woman has been taking pills for a protracted time without any days off, stop pills, wait 7 days, and start a new cycle.
9. Absence of withdrawal menses
a. Obtain history regarding absence of slight spotting, missed pills, pregnancy symptoms, nipple discharge.
b. Determine if woman has been taking pills for a protracted time without any days off. If so, stop pills for 7 days.
c. Rule out pregnancy.
d. Change to a pill with a progestin of higher endometrial activity (Lo-Ovral, Ovcon 35, or Nordette), or increase estrogen potency by changing to a more estrogenic active 35 µg pill or increasing estrogen dose up to 50 µg[3]

G. Teaching
1. Inform woman of noncontraceptive benefits of combined oral contraceptives.[13]
a. Decreased incidence of pelvic inflammatory disease
b. Decreased risk of endometrial and ovarian cancer
c. Decreased hospitalization for functional ovarian cysts
d. Less dysmenorrhea and decreased menstrual blood loss
e. Decreased fibrocystic breast disease
f. Less rheumatoid arthritis
2. Inform woman that use-effectiveness of oral contraceptives is 98-99 percent.
3. Review warning signs *(ACHES)* of oral contraceptives, and give the woman written material of these emphasizing the importance of immediately notifying the provider if they occur[7]:
a. Abdominal pain: a sign of hepatic adenoma or gallbladder disease
b. Chest pain or shortness of breath: a sign of embolism or myocardial infarction, which is usually preceded by repeated episodes of severe chest pain

    c. Headaches (severe): a sign of impending stroke or (more rarely) hypertension

    d. Eye problems, including blurred vision or loss of vision: a sign of hypertension

    e. Severe leg pains: a sign of thromboembolism

4. Have the woman take a pill every day at the same time each day.

5. For first three cycles, the woman should record on a calendar any side effects, including breakthrough bleeding, edema, acne, and withdrawal bleeding.

6. Alert the woman she may have breakthrough bleeding during first three to four cycles.

7. Have woman utilize another form of contraception for the first pill cycle.

8. Advise woman to eat a well-balanced diet and take a daily multivitamin supplement.

9. Give specific instructions regarding missed pills, prolonged diarrhea, or vomiting.

10. Ask woman to return for refill prior to finishing her pack.

11. When woman is seen for a medical problem, she should tell the practitioner she is taking OCPs.

12. Instruct woman to call a provider if minor side effects occur.

III. Steroidal contraceptives: progestin only

A. History

    1. Absolute contraindications (see Section II, A, 1)

Undiagnosed uterine bleeding is an important contraindication since irregular menses are a side effect.

---

    2. Relative contraindications[7]

        a. Active mononucleosis

        b. Ectopic pregnancy history

        c. History of irregular menses

        d. History of gestational diabetes

B. Physical assessment

    1. Obtain baseline weight.

    2. Take blood pressure.

    3. Perform pelvic exam with Pap smear.

C. Laboratory studies

    1. Obtain lipid screen if at high risk for cardiovascular disease.

    2. Obtain glucose tolerance test if at risk for carbohydrate intolerance (e.g., family history or history of gestational diabetes).

D. Management of progestin pill therapy

    1. Profile of a good candidate for progestin-only pills:

        a. Woman who must change from combined pills due to complications or side effects.

b. Woman with relative contraindications for combined pills, including severe varicosities and history of migraine headaches.

c. Woman who is lactating.

2. Women who cannot tolerate irregular menses are not good candidates.

3. Obtain signed informed consent from patient regarding the risks and benefits.

4. Prescribe three to six cycles of pills.

5. Evaluate blood pressure and any problems after initial prescription.

6. If no problems after initial prescription, provide a 7-month supply.

7. Schedule woman for annual exam.

8. Repeat lipid screen or obtain liver function studies as indicated since progestin can alter these serum levels.

E. Teaching

1. Inform woman that use-effectiveness of progestin-only pills is 96-98 percent.

2. Inform woman of noncontraceptive benefits.

a. Decreased dysmenorrhea

b. Decreased incidence of pelvic inflammatory disease

3. Woman must know warning signs of complications (see Sec. II. G. 3).

4. Woman should take one pill every day continuously without interruption. This is important to stress to women switching from the combination pill.

5. Woman should also use another form of contraception for the first two cycles.

6. Inform woman she may have irregular menses and/or spotting.

7. If no menses for 45 days, woman should have a pregnancy test.

8. Continuation of regular menses may indicate ovulatory cycles. Woman should be encouraged to utilize another method at midcycle (days 10-18).

9. Provide specific instructions regarding missed pills, prolonged diarrhea, or vomiting.

10. When seen for a medical problem, woman should inform the practitioner she is taking progestin-only pills.

Practitioners should attempt to avoid using the term minipill *since many patients confuse progestin-only pills with low-dose combined oral contraceptives.*

F. Management of side effects: progestins contribute to the following side effects (since progestin-only pills have less progestin than combination pills, it is expected that these side effects would be less frequent and less severe):

1. Increased level of high-density lipoproteins[10]

a. Screen as appropriate.

b. Encourage woman to alter diet to limit excess saturated fat, sugar, and calories.

2. Changes in carbohydrate metabolism

a. Obtain a diet history.

b. Suggest alterations in diet to maintain ideal weight.

c. Encourage moderate exercise program.

    3. Hypertension
       Discontinue hormonal contraceptives and change to nonhormonal contraceptive.
    4. Acne or oily skin
       a. Encourage use of drying agents (e.g., benzoyl peroxide), or refer to dermatologist.
       b. Change to nonhormonal contraceptive if condition worsens.
    5. Depression and decreased libido
       a. Assure diet adequate in vitamin B_6 (25 mg daily).
       b. Change to nonhormonal contraceptive or combined hormonal contraceptive.
    6. Hirsutism: discontinue pill.
    7. Edema: discontinue pill.
    8. Change in liver function tests: discontinue pill.
  G. Other routes of administering progestins
    1. Long-acting progestin injection: Depo-Provera is most commonly used: however, not approved for use in the United States
    2. Norplant subdermal implants
       a. Six silastic capsules are implanted containing levonorgestrel, which provides 5 years of contraception once implanted.[9]
       b. FDA approval is pending.
       c. Side effects are similar to those of the progestin pill.
       d. Implants require minor surgical procedure to insert and remove.
    3. Future possibilities
       a. IUD with a slow-released progestin effective for 5 years
       b. Contraceptive vaginal ring with progestin worn for 21 days

IV. Intrauterine devices (may become limited in the United States due to the withdrawal of all types except the Progestasert)

A. History
    1. Absolute contraindications are as follows[7]:
       a. Active pelvic infection
       b. Known or suspected pregnancy
    2. Relative contraindications are as follows[7]:
       a. Recent or recurrent pelvic infection
       b. Multiple sex partners
       c. Purulent cervicitis
       d. History of an ectopic pregnancy
       e. Impaired response to infection (diabetes or steroid treatment)
       f. Presence of abnormal uterine bleeding
       g. Concern about future fertility especially if previous pelvic infection
    3. Other important aspects of the history include the following:
       a. Menstrual history
          • Regularity
          • Length of menses

- Flow
- Dysmenorrhea
  b. Gynecological history
  - History of abnormal Pap smear
  c. Medical history
  - Anemia
  - Clotting disorders
  - Subbacterial endocarditis history due to increase in possibility of infection
B. Physical assessment (perform bimanual exmination to determine uterine position and to rule out infection or pregnancy)
  1. Caution should be exercised in inserting an IUD if the woman has a retroflexed uterus
  2. A postpartum uterus less than 8 weeks may be perforated more easily.
C. Laboratory studies (prior to insertion)
  1. Pap for cancer and actinomyses diagnosis
  2. *Gonorrhea* culture
  3. *Chlamydia* test as appropriate
  4. Wet mount as appropriate
  5. Hemoglobin or hematocrit
  6. Pregnancy test if unprotected coitus prior to insertion
D. Management of minor complications
  1. Spotting, bleeding, anemia
    a. Progestasert IUD may lessen these side effects
    b. Rule out other causes: PID, partial expulsion, cancer, polyps, postcoital spotting.
    c. Provide iron supplement if slight to moderate anemia.
    d. If blood loss causes significant anemia, remove IUD and provide alternative contraception.
  2. Cramping and pain
    a. During insertion, sound slowly and gently.
    b. After insertion do the following:
      - Severe: remove IUD; if vasovagal response, give atropine subcutaneously.
      - Mild: give aspirin or antiprostaglandin medication.
  3. IUD expulsion
    a. Symptoms
      - Cramping or pain
      - Unusual vaginal discharge
      - Intermenstrual or postcoital spotting.
      - Dyspareunia
      - IUD felt in the os
    b. Complete explusion: first indication may be a missed period, missing strings, or early pregnancy symptoms
    c. Partial expulsion

- Remove IUD
- Replace IUD immediately if no contraindications.
  4. Lost strings
     a. Examine vagina for strings; usually they can be visualized although woman cannot palpate them. Teach woman to palpate them correctly.
     b. Probe cervical canal gently for strings with narrow forceps.
     c. Perform pregnancy test if above are negative.
     d. Use ultrasound or radiography to visualize IUD and assist in removal from uterine cavity.
  5. Difficult removal
     a. Remove IUD during menses.
     b. Use of paracervical block and cervical dilators may be necessary.
     c. If no strings visible, probe canal with narrow forceps.
E. Management of serious complications
  1. Pelvic inflammatory disease: prevention strategies
     a. *Gonorrhea neisseria*
        - Remove IUD when diagnosed.
        - If present prior to insertion, treat first.
     b. *Chlamydia*
        - Woman should be free of *Chlamydia* for 6 months before insertion.
        - If IUD in place, treat and do not remove unless PID symptoms are present.
     c. *Actinomyces*
        - If IUD in place and woman is asymptomatic, treat with tetracycline and do not remove IUD; repeat Pap in 3-4 months.
        - If woman is symptomatic, remove IUD and treat.
  2. Uterine or cervical perforation or embedding
     a. Woman may be symptomatic or asymptomatic.
     b. Ultrasound is effective in locating IUD.
     c. Refer to physician if symptoms are causing problems.
  3. Pregnancy
     a. There is an increased risk of sepsis, especially if strings are visible.
     b. There is a 50 percent chance of spontaneous abortion if IUD is left in place versus 25 percent if IUD is removed.[14]
F. Follow-up management (at 6 weeks)
  1. Ascertain presence of danger signs or side effects.
  2. Check hemoglobin or hematocrit, if heavy menses are reported.
  3. Visualize strings and trim if too long-especially with Copper-7.
  4. Perform wet mount and/or culture if abnormal discharge or cervicitis present.
  5. Reschedule for annual exam.
G. Teaching
  1. Inform woman of noncontraceptive benefits: Progestasert IUD results in less menstrual bleeding and less dysmenorrhea.
  2. Teach woman to feel for IUD strings.

3. Instruct her to check for her strings weekly for the first 2 months and then after each menses.
4. Give woman a card with the name of the IUD she has and information regarding replacement.
   a. Progestasert: replace every year
   b. Copper devices: replace every 4 years
   c. Nonmedicated devices: indefinite placement
5. Instruct in the use of alternative contraceptive method for 4-8 weeks.
6. Plan return visit in 6 weeks to check strings.
7. Teach danger signs (*PAINS*) which are as follows[7]:
   a. *P*eriod: late, with abnormal spotting or bleeding
   b. *A*bdominal pain and pain with intercourse
   c. *I*nfection exposure (e.g., gonorrhea) or abnormal discharge
   d. *N*ot feeling well: fever and chills
   e. *S*tring missing: shorter or longer.
8. Review expected immediate side effects and cautions.
   a. Cramping and spotting for 1-2 days
      • Suggest antiprostaglandin medication (e.g., Ibuprofen) every 4 hours for pain.
      • Pain, bleeding, or discharge persisting greater than a few days may be indicative of a pelvic infection.
   b. No sexual intercourse for 24-48 hours postinsertion
   c. May take 3 months to adjust to IUD
      • Woman may have heavier or longer periods than preinsertion.
      • Woman may have cramping or increased dysmenorrhea.
      • Explain to woman that the kind of menses she has by the third month is predictive of future menses.
9. Review lost IUD string instructions.
   a. More likely to occur during menses, so check pads, tampons, and toilet at this time.
   b. If having cramping, check for strings.
   c. If unable to feel strings or if IUD is felt in the os:
      • Make an appointment to be checked.
      • Use another form of contraception until appointment.
10. If desiring pregnancy, remove IUD 3 months prior to pregnancy.
11. If pregnant with IUD, have it removed if the strings are visible.
12. If a period is missed or pregnancy is possible, woman should see her practitioner immediately.
13. Tell woman to inform her practitioner that she has an IUD if she is seen for a medical, surgical, or sexual problem.

V. Diaphragm

A. History
   1. History of toxic shock syndrome (contraindication)
   2. Allergy to latex and/or spermicidal preparation

3. Abnormalities of the vagina (uterine prolapse, severe anteversion or retroversion, fistulas): will not permit good fit.
4. Prior use: successful versus unsuccessful and why

B. Physical assessment
   1. Assess vaginal musculature for tone, prolapse, cystocele, or rectocele.
   2. Assess pelvic architecture, i.e., depth of retropubic angle.
   3. Determine severe ante- or retroflexion.
   4. Measure the length from the posterior fornix to the symphysis pubis.

C. Laboratory studies (obtain wet mount, if appropriate)

D. Initial mangement
   1. Choose a diaphragm.
      a. Arcing spring rim: provides firm spring strength, which may be needed with fair or poor vaginal tone.
      b. Coil spring rim: provides similar spring strength as arcing diaphragm. When folded, maintains a flat configuration for insertion.
      c. Flat spring rim: a delicate, thin rim. Provides gentle strength. Preferred for women with firm vaginal tone and a shallow arch.
      d. Wide seal rim: a diaphragm with a 1.5-cm-wide seal in the inner rim to keep spermicide in the diaphragm and improve the seal between the vaginal walls. The diaphragm is available as either an arcing or coil spring.
   2. Fit the diaphragm.
      a. Fit the woman with the largest size that is comfortable. General guidelines are as follows:
         • Nulliparas: 65-75 (may change with intercourse)
         • Multiparas: 75-85
         • Grand multiparas: >85
      b. Use actual diaphragm for fitting; fitting rings do not represent actual placement.
      c. Diaphragm should fit snuggly behind the symphsis.
         • Fit is too small
            — If more than one finger space between rim and symphysis pubis
            — If it moves freely in the vagina.
         • Fit is too large
            — If it does not allow a fingertip between the rim and symphysis pubis
            — If edge of diaphragm bulges out of the introitus
            — If rim buckles against vaginal walls
            — If woman feels discomfort when it is in place, including abdominal cramping, backache, difficulty urinating, rectal pressure, or cramps in inner thighs
   3. Teach woman to insert diaphragm and check that her cervix is covered and rim is under retropubic arch.
   4. Check placement after insertion by woman.
   5. Teach woman to remove diaphragm (may use a Valsalva maneuver).

6. Inability of woman or partner to learn correct insertion or removal technique should result in an alternative contraceptive choice.

E. Follow-up management
   1. Woman should return in 1-2 weeks wearing the diaphragm.
   2. Obtain history.
      a. Use: problems with insertion and removal
      b. Satisfaction with method
      c. Partner's satisfaction
      d. Symptoms while in place
   3. Check for signs and symptoms of cystitis.[5]
   4. Check diaphragm for the following:
      a. Size
      b. Placement
      c. Presence of pelvic pain
      d. Presence of irritation

F. Teaching
   1. Inform the woman that the diaphragm works by holding the spermicide next to the cervix, not by acting as a barrier.[2]
   2. Inform woman that the effectiveness rate varies between 81 and 98 percent.
   3. Inform woman about the noncontraceptive benefits.
      a. Protection against sexually transmitted diseases[16]
      b. Decreased incidence of PID
      c. Decreased cervical dysplasia and/or cancer
   4. Discuss preparation and usage.
      a. Put 1-2 tablespoons of spermicide in center of diaphragm and around edges.
      b. Insert diaphragm up to 6 hours prior to intercourse.
      c. Check to see that cervix is covered and the rim is behind the symphysis after insertion and a bowel movement.
      d. Insert more spermicide vaginally if repeat coitus after 6 hours. Do not remove the diaphragm.
      e. Keep diaphragm in place for six hours after last coitus.
      f. Woman should not feel the diaphragm or experience low backache, abdominal cramping, inner thigh pain, or problems with voiding while wearing the diaphragm.
   5. Instruct in care of diaphragm.
      a. Wash with mild soap and dry.
      b. Store in plastic case.
      c. Check for holes or signs of puncturing.
      d. If the woman has had vaginitis, soak the diaphragm in 70 percent alcohol for 20 minutes to avoid reinfection.
   6. Instruct woman to have diaphragm refitted:
      a. If diaphragm no longer fits, e.g., if more than one fingertip can be introduced between the symphysis and rim or if buckling is noted.

Specific weight change recommendations have been omitted since they are not supported in the literature.[11]

    b. After a second trimester abortion, full-term pregnancy, or pelvic sur-
       gery.
    c. If woman experiences recurrent cystitis, which may be due to pressure
       of rim on the urethra.
 7. Teach woman preventive measures against urinary tract infection. [5]
 8. Teach woman danger signs of toxic shock syndrome (TSS).
    a. Fever > 101°F or 39°C.
    b. Diarrhea
    c. Vomiting
    d. Muscle aches
    e. Rash (like sunburn)
 9. Inform woman her risk of TSS is greatly reduced if diaphragm is worn for
    less than 24 hours.

VI. Vaginal sponge

A. History
   1. History of TSS (contraindication)
   2. Allergy to latex and/or spermicide
   3. Abnormalities of the vagina (uterine prolapse, severe anteversion or
      retroversion, fistulas)
   4. Delivery within last 6-8 weeks
B. Physical assessment unnecessary
C. Laboratory studies unnecessary
D. Teaching
   1. Inform woman that the vaginal sponge is impregnated with spermicide
      providing contraception for 24 hours once activated with water.
   2. Inform woman that vaginal sponges are an over-the-counter product.
   3. Inform woman that effectiveness rate is approximately the same as the
      diaphgram at 89-91 percent.[4]
   4. Discuss proper usage.
      a. Use the sponge every time there is intercourse.
      b. Sponge must be activated with water prior to insertion.
      c. Check placement after insertion to assure dimple side against cervix
         and string side against finger.
      d. To assure effectiveness, check placement before and after intercourse.
         If sponge is displaced, woman may need to choose an alternative
         method.
      e. Do not use the sponge during menses (to decrease risk of TSS).
      f. Do not use the sponge to absorb abnormal vaginal discharge.
   5. Teach woman danger signs of TSS (see Section V, F, 7).
   6. Inform woman her risk of TSS is similar to that of a tampon user.

7. Discuss with woman that the presence of vulvar erythema may be due to sensitivity to spermicide.
8. Inform woman that 6 percent of users may have difficulty removing the sponge, resulting in tearing or requiring medical assistance.
E. Follow-up unnecessary except for difficulty with removal

VII. Cervical cap

Cervical caps are not currently approved for marketing in the United States, but they may be available at some research sites such as women's health centers.

A. History
   1. History of TSS (contraindication)
   2. Abnormality of the cervix resulting in poor fit
   3. Allergy to latex and/or spermicide
   4. Acute cervicitis or pelvic inflammatory disease
   5. Cervical biopsy or cryosurgery within 6 weeks
B. Physical assessment
   1. Rule out acute cervicitis.
   2. Assess cervix and vagina for abnormalities interfering with a good fit.
C. Laboratory studies
   1. Obtain wet mount as appropriate.
   2. Obtain cervical cultures as appropriate.
D. Management
   1. Fit the cap snugly to maintain suction between rim and cervix.
   2. Choose a cervical cap.
      a. Prentif cervical cap
         • Small, flexible, deep cap made of rubber with firm rim to provide good suction
         • Four sizes: 22 mm, 24 mm, 28 mm, and 31 mm
         • Good for a woman with long cervix
      b. Vimule cap
         • Shallow rubber cup: clings to vaginal vault instead of the cervix
         • Three sizes: 42 mm, 48 mm, and 54 mm
         • May cause lesions of portio vaginalis
      c. Dumas cap
         • Shallow rubber cap: fits similar to a small diaphragm
         • Four sizes: 50 mm, 55 mm, 60 mm, and 70 mm
         • May be used if flush or short cervix is present
   3. Inability of woman to learn correct insertion or removal technique should result in an alternative contraceptive choice.
E. Follow-up management (see Section V, E: all information applies except increased incidence of cystitis)
F. Teaching
   1. Inform woman the use-effectiveness rate varies between 80 and 95 percent although controlled studies are not yet available.

2. Noncontraceptive benefits are not well known, but caps probably provide some protection against STDs.
3. Instruct woman to fill cap one third full with spermicide prior to insertion.
4. Cap must remain in place 6-8 hours after intercourse.
5. If cap is left in during the entire intermenstrual period, woman may experience a malodorous discharge.
6. See provider if malodorous discharge does not clear after douching with clear water.
7. Remove cap during menses to avoid risk of TSS.

VIII. Barrier method: condom

A. History
   1. Ascertain if male is unable to maintain an erection.
   2. Elicit allergy to latex or spermicide.
B. Teaching
   1. Inform woman and/or partner of noncontraceptive benefits.
      a. Helps prevent STDs[16]
      b. May be used to help certain sexual dysfunctions, including premature ejaculation and inability to maintain an erection
      c. May prevent antibody response to sperm in couples with an infertility history
   2. Inform woman and/or partner of the following:
      a. Use-effectiveness rate is 90-95 percent.
      b. Efficacy is increased if used in conjunction with vaginal spermicide.
   3. Discuss types of condoms.
      a. Plain
      b. Lubricated
      c. Textured
      d. Mentor: thin, lubricated sheath with light adhesive at the base to prevent accidental removal after coitus
   4. Discuss usage and removal.
      a. Apply condom to an erect penis prior to vaginal penetration.
      b. After coitus, hold condom at base during removal of the penis in order to avoid spilling sperm in the vagina.
      c. Remove the condom away from the vagina.
      d. Do not reuse a condom.
   5. Discuss proper storage of new condoms (away from excessive heat—e.g., hip pocket, glove compartments—which may damage latex and predispose to breakage)

IX. Natural family planning methods (fertility awareness methods)

A. Calendar method
   1. Contraception is obtained by abstaining during the time of ovulation.

2. Relative contraindications are the following:
    a. Very short menstrual cycles
    b. Highly variable menstrual cycles
3. Management and teaching
    a. Record 6-12 consecutive menstrual cycles.
    b. Subtract 18 from shortest cycle: first fertile day.
    c. Subtract 11 from longest cycle: last fertile day.
    d. Abstain from intercourse during period of first to last fertile day. Example: if short cycle is 24 days and long cycle is 32 days then woman should abstain from day 6 through day 21 of the cycle.
B. Basal body temperature method
    1. Identify ovulation by body temperature elevation. Once a temperature elevation of 0.4-0.8°F has been noted for 3 consecutive days, the woman may safely have intercourse until the beginning of her next cycle.
    2. Warn woman of conditions that can disturb body temperature:
        a. Large alcohol intake
        b. Sleeplessness
        c. GI or other illness
        d. Immunization
        e. Warm or hot climate
        f. Use of an electric blanket
    3. Provide management and teaching.
        a. Use a basal temperature thermometer to obtain accurate readings.
        b. Teach woman to take her temperature for 5 minutes every morning before getting out of bed or doing any activity—including smoking.
        c. Woman should record her temperature on graph paper (with 0.1 markings) and connect readings to obtain baseline temperature reading.
        d. At ovulation, her temperature will rise 0.4-0.8°F above her baseline preovulatory level.
        e. Some women notice a drop in temperature 24 hours prior to ovulation.
        f. Once the 0.4-0.8°F rise has been noted for three consecutive days, woman can safely resume intercourse. Intercourse prior to this time can result in accidental pregnancy.
        g. These are only basic instructions; couples relying on this method should be referred to trained counselors.
C. Mucus method (Billings)
    1. Ovulation can be identified by cervical and mucus changes that occur during the menstrual cycle.
    2. The main relative contraindication is a woman uncomfortable touching herself.
    3. Management and teaching are as follows:
        a. Pre- and postovulatory mucus is yellow, viscous, and dry.
        b. Ovulatory mucus is slippery and clear, like egg whites and can be stretched between two fingers (spinnbarkeit).
        c. Advise woman to check her vagina each day, noting the presence of

mucus and its consistency and color and recording information on a special chart.

  d. Woman should refrain from intercourse if any mucus is present.

  e. Peak mucus is very clear, slippery, and stretchy and indicates ovulation.

  f. Four days after the peak mucus or when it has returned to dry, thick, and cloudy, woman may resume intercourse.

  g. Woman should record several cycles of the mucus changes to become familiar with her pattern before utilizing this method.

  h. Presence and consistency of mucus may be obscured by vaginal infection, vaginal medication, douching, and sexual arousal or semen.

  i. A woman should be referred to a trained counselor before utilizing this method.

D. Symptothermal method

  1. Uses cervical, cervical mucus, and basal body temperature changes simultaneously as indicators of ovulation.

  2. Management and teaching must integrate components of all three methodologies.

X. Postcoital contraception

A. History

  1. Date of last menstrual period

  2. Time of unprotected coitus

  3. Absence of absolute contraindications for oral contraceptives or IUD as appropriate (see Sections II, A and IV, A).

B. Physical examination (perform as applicable to rule out contraindications)

C. Laboratory studies (obtain a pregnancy test if indicated by history or exam)

D. Management and teaching

  1. Combined oral contraceptives[7]

    a. Use of Ovral pills is 98.5 percent effective in preventing pregnancy if given within 72 hours (preferably within 12-24 hours) of unprotected coitus.

    b. Tell woman to take two Ovral pills within 72 hours of unprotected coitus. Take two more Ovral pills 12 hours after first dose.

    c. Inform woman she may have nausea, which will resolve 24-48 hours after treatment.

      • If she vcmits within 1 hour of pill ingestion, she should contact her provider.

      • Provider may also need to prescribe antinausea medication.

    d. Make sure woman knows danger signs of oral contraceptives (see Section II, G, 3).

    e. Inform woman she can expect a period within 3 weeks. If she does not have a period after 3 weeks, she should contact her provider for a pregnancy test.

    f. Discuss with woman more long-term contraceptive options and stress that this method is a one-time-only method.

2. IUD
   a. Postcoital insertion of an IUD prevents implantation of a fertilized ovum and is nearly 100 percent effective.
   b. Insertion should occur within 5-7 days of unprotected coitus.
   c. Woman must know danger signs and side effects of the IUD (see Section IV).

REFERENCES

1. Bernstein G, Kilzer L, Coulson A, et al: Studies of cervical caps: I. Vaginal lesions associated with use of the Vimule cap. Contraception, 26(5):443-446, 1983
2. Bracken M: Spermicidal contraceptives and poor reproductive outcomes: The epidemiologic evidence against an association. Am J Obstet Gynecol 151:552-556, 1984
3. Dickey R: Managing Contraceptive Pill Patients (ed 4). Durant, OK, Creative Informatics, 1984
4. Edelman D, McIntyre S, Harper J: A comparative trial of the Today contraceptive sponge and diaphragm. Am J Obstet Gynecol 150:869-876, 1984
5. Fihn S, Johnson C, Pinkstaff G, Stamm W: Diaphragm use and urinary tract infections: Analysis of urodynamic and microbiological factors. J Urol 136(4):853-856, 1986
6. Fogel C, Woods N: Health Care of Women: A Nursing Perspective. St. Louis, Mosby, 1981
7. Hatcher R, Stewart F, Stewart G, et al: Contraceptive Technology, 1986-1987 (ed 13). New York, Irvington Press, 1986
8. Johnson J: The cervical cap: A retrospective study of an alternative contraceptive technique. Am J Obstet Gynecol 148:604-608, 1984
9. Kaufman D, Watson J, Rosenberg L, et al: The effect of different types of intrauterine devices on the risk of pelvic inflammatory disease. JAMA 250(6):759-762, 1983
10. Krauss R, Roy S, Mishell D, et al: Effects of two low-dose oral contraceptives on serum lipids and lipoproteins: Differential changes in high-density lipoprotein subclasses. Am J Obstet Gynecol 145:446-452, 1983
11. Kugel C, Verson H: Relationship between weight change and diaphragm size change. JOGN Nurse 15(2):123-129, 1986
12. Martin P: Handbook of Office Gynecology. Orlando, FL, Grune & Stratton, 1985
13. Ory H: The noncontraceptive health benefits from oral contraceptive use. Fam Plann Perspect 14:182-184, 1982
14. Perlmatter J: Pregnancy and the IUD. J Reprod Med 20:133, 1978
15. Speroff L, Glass R, Kase N: Clinical Gynecologic Endocrinology and Infertility (ed 3). Baltimore, Williams & Wilkins, p 1983

16. Stone K, Grimes D, Magder L: Personal protection against sexually transmit-
    ted diseases. Am J Obstet Gynecol 155(1):180-188, 1986
17. Tri-Norinyl and Ortho-Norum 7-7-7 Two triphasic oral contraceptives. Med
    Lett 26:93-94, 1984

Chapter 4

Care of the Menopausal Woman

Mary K. Barger

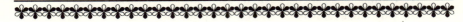

I. Purpose of visits

A. Evaluate for presence of menopause-related signs and symptoms.

B. Identify risk factors for osteoporosis.

C. Institute preventive measures for osteoporosis.

D. Teach woman preventive measures for common symptoms of menopause.

E. Provide an opportunity for woman to discuss feelings about body image, emotional changes, lifestyle changes, and sexuality with increasing age.

F. Perform a physical exam to screen for coincident medical or gynecological disease.

G. Institute hormone replacement therapy when appropriate, including patient education for rationale and side effects.

II. Menopause evaluation and management

A. History
1. Family history
   a. Coronary artery disease
   b. Breast cancer
   c. Osteoporosis (especially in woman's mother)
2. Personal history
   a. Cardiovascular problems and/or hypertension
   b. Breast disorders
   c. Liver disease or tumors
   d. Gallbladder disease
   e. Uterine disorders, including endometrial cancer, fibroids, previous abnormal Pap, and history of abnormal vaginal bleeding
   f. Insulin-dependent diabetes
3. Woman's impression of her physical condition including
   a. Presence of hot flushes
   b. Night sweats
   c. Insomnia

     d. Vaginal itching and irritation or dyspareunia.
     e. Urinary tract symptoms
  4. Woman's current physical status
     a. Possibility of pregnancy
     b. Presence of abnormal vaginal bleeding

Cervicovaginal cytology is inadequate to rule out malignancy. Patient must be referred for endometrial biopsy.

---

     c. Current medications, cigarette use, and alcohol intake
     d. Ongoing treatment for other health problems
B. Physical assessment
  1. Height (loss of height may be indicative of compression fractures or osteoporosis.)
  2. Weight
  3. Vital signs: blood pressure, pulse, and respirations
  4. Physical assessment
     a. Thyroid: disorder may be responsible for menopausal-like or osteoporotic-like symptoms
     b. Heart: rule out cardiovascular disease
     c. Lungs: rule out existing respiratory disease
     d. Breasts: presence of masses or nipple discharge
     e. Abdomen: masses
     f. Extremities: edema or varicosities
     g. Genitourinary tract:
       • Assess vagina for signs of atrophy.
       • Assess vaginal muscle tone, and presence of cystocele or rectocele.
       • Pap smear must adequately sample the squamocolumnar junction, which often recedes into cervical canal.
       • Refer to physician if any adnexae are palpated.
     h. Rectum: polyps, other masses.
C. Laboratory tests
  1. Complete blood count: yearly
  2. Blood lipids: yearly or as necessary
  3. Liver function: prior to hormone replacement therapy
  4. Pap smear (for posthysterectomy women, take specimen from vaginal cuff and vaginal pool): yearly
  5. Stool specimen for occult blood: yearly
D. Management and teaching with normal findings
  1. During perimenopause, women must continue to use contraception to avoid pregnancy.
  2. Until cessation of menses, pregnancy must be ruled out as a cause of amenorrhea.
  3. Continued, regular sexual activity is helpful in the prevention of atrophic vaginitis.[5]

4. Kegel exercises, 50-100 every day, should be done to strengthen pubococcygeus muscle and minimize urinary tract problems.
5. As part of nutrition counseling, explain that the following dietary changes will help counteract any tendency to gain weight:
   a. Reduction in salt
   b. Reduction in animal fats
   c. Adequate intake of all nutrients over three meals a day
   d. Decrease in calories if woman is overweight or increase if underweight
6. Teach measures useful in the prevention of osteoporosis, compression fractures, and hip fractures.[13,17]
   a. Recommend calcium intake adequate to prevent bone loss, either 1000 mg elemental calcium per day if on hormone therapy or 1500 mg elemental calcium per day if not taking hormones.
      • Average diet contains 400 mg elemental calcium each day.
      • Eight ounces of milk contains 300 mg of elemental calcium.
      • Calcium carbonate contains 400 mg of elemental calcium per 1000 mg. (Least expensive source is Tums: contains 200 mg elemental calcium per tablet.)
      • Calcium lactate contains 130 mg elemental calcium in 1000 mg.
      • Calcium gluconate contains 10 mg elemental calcium in 1000 mg.
   b. Diet should not be excessive in fiber, protein, or carbohydrate, all of which may interfere with calcium absorption.
   c. Encourage woman to stop smoking.
   d. Encourage woman to decrease caffeine and alcohol intake.
   e. Recommend regular amount of weight-bearing exercise, such as walking.[10]
   f. Minimize the use of drugs that interfere with calcium absorption:
      • Anticonvulsants such as Dilantin
      • Corticosteroids
      • Tetracycline
      • Isoniazid
      • "Loop" diuretics
      • Antacids containing aluminum
   g. Consider hormone replacement therapy, especially if woman is at high risk even though currently asymptomatic.
7. Instruct woman to return to care provider for treatment if the following symptoms occur or increase in severity:
   a. Hot flushes or night sweats
   b. Headaches
   c. Nausea
   d. Palpitations
   e. Dizziness
   f. Vaginal itching or irritation or dyspareunia
   g. Urinary symptoms, including frequency, pain, urgency, and incontinence

  h. Insomnia
  i. Depression, fatigue, and/or libido changes
  8. Teach or review breast self-exam.
E. Management of abnormal findings
  1. Hot flushes or night sweats[16]
    a. Prescribe hormone replacement therapy (HRT) (see Section III).
    b. An alternative treatment is to prescribe clonidine hydrochloride 1/10 mg tab: cut in one quarter and take PO TID.[15]
    c. Increase vitamin E in diet: food sources are peanuts, soybeans, spinach, wheat germ, and vegetable oils.
    d. Assure adequate vitamin B complex in diet: food sources are whole grains, yogurt, wheat germ, liver, and brewer's yeast.
  2. Atrophic vaginitis
    a. Prescribe hormone replacement therapy.
    b. Apply estrogen vaginally:
      • Conjugated estrogen cream: one half of an applicator one to two times per week, or
      • Estradiol tablet vaginally twice weekly

Estrogen administered vaginally is absorbed systemically; therefore, follow the guidelines for oral estrogen (see Section III).

---

    c. Use exogenous lubrication, such as Transi-Lube foam, especially during intercourse.
  3. Urinary symptoms
    a. Urinary atrophy may be avoided with HRT or vaginal estrogen.
    b. Assess for presence of cystocele or urethrocele and degree and refer if surgery indicated.
  4. Psychological changes and mood change, emotional lability, depression, and melancholy[5]
    a. Menopausal symptoms have historically been attributed mostly to psychological causes, e.g., "loss of femininity," or "the empty nest syndrome." The reality may be much different for women who are in satisfactory careers, finally feel free of becoming pregnant, and look forward to quiet without having to care for children. These women's greatest obstacle may be the perceptions of others, including dealing with stereotypes of older women and male partners' perceptions of the effect of menopause.
    b. Ascertain if patient is depressed: use a self-rating scale (e.g., Beck Depression Inventory) plus history. One study showed that 45 percent of women rated normal on a self-rating depression scale although others were telling them they were depressed.[7]
    c. If patient is depressed, initiate HRT, which may resolve the depression rapidly. If depression is not relieved within 1 month, refer for appropriate therapy.

    d. If there is a problem with others' perception, refer for family therapy.

    e. Stress reduction techniques may be helpful.

III. Hormone replacement therapy (HRT)[5]

A. Definition: exogenous replacement of estrogen and progesterone to alleviate menopausal symptoms or prevent osteoporosis[8]

B. Benefits
    1. Decreases severity and frequency of vasomotor symptoms
    2. Often improves woman's mood
    3. Decreases genitourinary atrophy[15]
    4. Decreases severity or prevents osteoporosis[1,4,14]
        a. Assists absorption of calcium and prevents its excretion
        b. Stimulates calcitonin
        c. Blocks the effect of bone-reabsorbing parathyroid hormone
        d. Inhibits breakdown of old bone
    5. Increases formation of liver hormones
    6. Decreases atherosclerosis by altering serum lipoprotein to a lower risk profile[1,2,9] (documented for estrogen only; unclear if benefit remains when used with progestin[1])
    7. Decreases risk of myocardial infarction and incidence of symptomatic atherosclerosis[2,9]
    8. Does not increase risk of thromboembolism, stroke, or heart disease at current doses[2]

C. Disadvantages

Use of exogenous estrogen without progestin increases incidence of endometrial cancer.[1]

---

    1. Increases risk of gallbladder disease two to five times.
    2. Side effects include the following:
        a. Breast tenderness
        b. Nausea
        c. Edema
        d. Breakthrough bleeding
        e. Stimulation of fibroids

D. Contraindications
    1. History or presence of estrogen-dependent neoplasm[6,11]
    2. Presence of undiagnosed vaginal bleeding
    3. History of or current presence of thromboembolism.
    4. Presence of active or severe liver disease
    5. Woman unresponsive to education

E. Relative contraindications
    1. Insulin-dependent diabetes
    2. Gallbladder disease
    3. Uterine fibroids or endometriosis

F. Administration[12]
  1. Selection
    a. If the woman is estrogen deficient, use lowest dose to relieve estrogen-deficient symptoms.
    b. If the woman is at high risk for osteoporosis, use 0.625-mg conjugated estrogen or equivalent (see Section IV).
  2. Dosage schedule

Nonphysician providers should consult with a physician prior to ordering the following or act according to state statutes regarding prescribing drugs according to a standardized formulary.

---

    a. Estrogen taken days 1-26 each calendar month:
       conjugated estrogen, 0.625 mg;
         or
       estradiol, 1 mg;
         or
       ethinyl estradiol, 0.02 mg;
         or
       mestranol 0.2 mg;
         plus
       progestin, taken days 16 (or 19)-25 each calendar month:
       medroxyprogesterone acetate, 10 mg;
         or
       norethindrone acetate, 5 mg.
    b. No hormones are taken for the remainder of the month.
    c. Although this schedule is essential for women who have a uterus, controversy remains whether progestins are desirable for those women without a uterus.[1]
  3. Follow-up
    a. Visits should be scheduled every 3 months until the woman is regulated or a minimum dose to treat symptoms is achieved.
    b. Duration of hormone replacement therapy may be variable and dependent on symptoms or indefinite if prescribed for prevention of genital atrophy or osteoporosis.
  4. Education
    a. Make sure woman clearly understands both why she is undergoing HRT and also understands the ancillary benefits of the therapy.
    b. Explain physiology of withdrawal bleeding and assure acceptance of this side effect.
    c. Assure clear understanding of other common side effects and instruct woman to record them.
    d. Instruct woman to record frequency and duration of symptoms being treated.
    e. Make sure woman knows the signs of gallbladder disease, including abdominal pain, nausea and vomiting, anorexia, and jaundice.

5. Initiation of HRT

In some communities, the following two tests are recommended prior to initiation of therapy. However, some practitioners feel that in the absence of abnormal vaginal bleeding or high-risk factors, they are unnecessary.

   a. Endometrial biopsy
- By a physician as an office visit.
- To assess the condition of endometrium and presence of hyperplasia
- To rule out endometrial carcinoma
- At initiation of HRT, annually, and at termination of HRT

   b. Progesterone challenge test
- Progestin is given orally for 5-10 days and bleeding is noted.
- Withdrawal bleeding may be indicative of adequate endogenous estrogens to prevent osteoporosis; hence, HRT may not be necessary.

6. Management of side effects
   a. If breast tenderness and/or edema occurs, decrease estrogen dose.
   b. If nausea occurs, woman should do the following:
- Take dose before sleep
- Change to vaginal route of administration of estrogen (e.g., Estrace, 0.5-1.0 mg per vagina)—may avoid oral side effects with equivalent systemic levels

   c. Breakthrough bleeding: woman's report of this side effect is essential since it must be investigated. Refer woman to physician for endometrial biopsy.

IV. Osteoporosis

A. History[14]: risk factors
1. Family history of hip fracture, espcially woman's mother
2. Northern European ancestry
3. Age 60-70
4. Nulliparity
5. Premature menopause
6. Small stature and lean physique
7. Low physical activity level
8. Smoking
9. Excessive alcohol intake
10. Low calcium intake
11. Long-term use of corticosteroids or anticonvulsants
12. Gastric or small bowel resection
13. Hyperparathyroidism
14. Thyrotoxicosis

B. Physical exam
1. Observe for presence or absence of dowager's hump.
2. Observe if arms are too long compared with height.

3. Observe if woman walks with a limp.
4. Compare stature to height at younger age.
   a. Loss of height 1-2 in. may be present.
   b. Loss of height 3-8 in. is common if compression fractures are present.
C. Diagnostic laboratory studies (to be performed for a woman with a compression fracture):
   1. Serum tests: calcium, phosphorus, alkaline phosphatase
   2. Calcium and creatinine: 24-hour urine
   3. Bone mass quantitation: CT scan or single- or double-photon absorpitometry. Thirty-five percent bone loss is necessary before bone loss is noted via radiography. Photodensitometry of a single site, such as the wrist, is not diagnostic.
D. Differential diagnoses
   1. Hyperparathyroidism
   2. Multiple myeloma
   3. Cushing's syndrome
   4. Hyperthyroidism
   5. Osteomalacia (rare)
   6. Liver disease
   7. Malabsorption syndromes
   8. Osteogenesis imperfecta
   9. Increased calciuria
   10. Primary hypogonadism
   11. Alcoholism (leading cause of osteoporosis in men)
   12. Use of drugs interfering with calcium absorption or utilization (i.e., anticonvulsants, corticosteroids, heparin, antacids with aluminum)[5]
   13. Malignancy
E. Management and teaching
   1. Early postmenopausal women with decreased bone mass
      a. Follow guidelines for prevention (see Section II, D, 6).
      b. Start HRT at 0.625-mg conjugated estrogen dose.
      c. Order calcitonin-salmon injections, if woman has had a fracture. This treatment is expensive if given daily (approximately $200 a month). One center reports adequate treatment if given every 3 days with half the recommended dose.[3]
   2. Women who are already osteoporotic
      a. Continue to exercise.
      b. Intake 1000-1500 mg of calcium per day.
      c. Intake vitamin D, 400 IU per day (maximum dose 1000 IU per day).

REFERENCES

1. Barrett-Connor E: Postmenopausal estrogen, cancer and other considerations. Women Health 11(3/4):179-195, 1986
2. Bush T, Cowan L, Barrett-Connor E, et al: Estrogen use and all-cause mor-

tality: Preliminary results from the lipid research clinics program follow-up study. JAMA 249(7):903-906, 1983

3. Chestnut C: Presentation at UCSD School of Medicine, San Diego, 1986
4. Coralli C, Raisz L, Wood C: Osteoporosis: Significance, risk factors, and treatment. Nurse Pract 11(9):16-35, 1986
5. Cutler W, Garcia G: The Medical Mangagement of Menopause and Premenopause: Their Endocrinological Basis. Philadephia, JB Lippincott, 1984
6. Gambrell R, Maier R, Sanders B: Decreased incidence of breast cancer in postmenopausal estrogen-progestin users. Obstet Gynecol 62(4):435-443, 1983
7. Hamburger S: Presentation on first 100 women from UCSD Menopause Clinic, San Diego, 1986
8. Hammond C, Nachtigall L: Is estrogen therapy necessary? J Reprod Med 30(105):797-801, 1985
9. Henderson B, Ross R, Paganini-Hill A: Estrogen use and cardiovascular disease. J Reprod Med 30(105):814-820, 1985
10. Jensen J, Christiansen C, Rodbro P: Cigarette smoking, serum estrogens and bone loss during hormone replacement therapy early after menopause. N Engl J Med 313(16):973, 1985
11. Kaufman D, Miller D, Rosenberg L, et al: Noncontraceptive estrogen use and the risk of breast cancer. JAMA 252(1):63-67, 1984
12. Ladewig P: Protocol for estrogen replacement therapy in menopausal women. Nurse Pract 10(10):44-47, 1985
13. Marcus R: The relationship of dietary calcium to the maintenance of skeletal integrity in man—An interface of endocrinology and nutrition. Metabolism 31(1):93-102, 1982
14. Riggs B, Melton L: Involutional osteoporosis. N Engl J Med 314(26):1676-1684, 1986
15. Semmens J, Tsai C, Semmens C, et al: Effects of estrogen therapy on vaginal physiology during menopause. Obstet Gynecol 66(1):15-18, 1985
16. Tulandi T, Lal S: Menopausal hot flush. Obstet Gynecol Surv 40(9):553, 1985
17. White J: Osteoporosis: Strategies for prevention. Nurse Pract 11(9): 36-50, 1986

BIBLIOGRAPHY

Cutler W, Garcia G, Edwards D: Menopause: A guide for women and the men who love them. New York, WW Norton, 1983

Chapter 5

Antepartum Management

Judith T. Fullerton

I. Diagnosis of pregnancy

A. Purpose of the visit
   1. To confirm the state of pregnancy as the reason for amenorrhea
   2. To establish the gestational age of pregnancy by using Naegles rule (and by physical exam per protocol of the setting)
   3. To provide guidance and referral to sources of prenatal care
   4. To provide initial education regarding healthy pregnancy behaviors appropriate to the gestational age
B. History
   1. Pattern of menstrual cycles (regularity and amount of flow)
   2. First day of last normal menstrual period (LNMP)
   3. Type of contraceptives used (ever, and prior to the LNMP)
   4. Presumptive signs and symptoms of pregnancy
      a. Onset of amenorrhea
      b. Nausea and vomiting
      c. Quickening (first perception of fetal movement at 16-18 or 20 weeks, depending on parity)
      d. Sleep disturbance and associated fatigue
      e. Tingling, tenderness, and enlargement of the breasts with appearance of Montgomery's tubercles and color changes of the nipple
      f. Urinary frequency and/or urgency
      g. Weight change
      h. Elevation of the basal body temperature beyond 16-18 days after ovulation
C. Physical exam (see Section II, C)
D. Laboratory studies

Urine test accuracy is improved with a concentrated specimen, e.g., the first-voided morning urine.

---

1. Urine tests for pregnancy (in order of sensitivity)[8,10]
   a. Monoclonal urine: ICON HCG (Hybritech)
      • This is 100 percent accurate at 50 miu/ml. HCG is equivalent to day 1 of the first missed period (may also detect smaller concentrations).
      • Results can be obtained in 6-7 minutes.
   b. Slide test (ultrasensitive): Sensi-slide (Roche) or UCG-Beta Slide (Wampole)
      • More than 98 percent accurate at time of first missed period or following
      • Results in 2 minutes
   c. Slide tests (routine): Prognosticon or UCG Slide Test
      • More than 98 percent accurate 10-14 days from first missed period (only slightly less accurate at 5 days from first missed period)
      • Results in 2 minutes
   d. Hemagglutination inhibition tube test: home pregnancy tests including E-P-T, Daisy 2; and Gravidex (Ortho)
      • Results are 98 percent accurate at 10-14 days from first missed period
      • Results obtained in 30-90 minutes
2. Serum tests for pregnancy
   a. Radioimmunoassay (RIA) tests
      • Have the highest sensitivity and accuracy of all tests. Detects HCG at 8-10 days postconception.
      • Results obtained in 1-3 hours. (Many laboratories will only process several samples at a time; therefore, results may be delayed.)
   b. Radioreceptor (RRA) test
      • This is highly accurate 10-14 days postconception, but it cannot distinguish between HCG and luteinizing hormone.
      • Results can be obtained in 1 hour.
E. Teaching if exam is positive for pregnancy
   1. Assess woman's feelings about the pregnancy: allow for initial ambivalence.
   2. Discuss pregnancy options as appropriate.
   3. Discuss value of early and continuing prenatal care and provide referral to the variety of providers and settings.
   4. Inform woman of health behaviors that can adversely affect the pregnancy (e.g., alcohol, tobacco, and drug use).
   5. Discuss the false-positive and false-negative risk of laboratory examinations, as appropriate to gestational age and type of test used for diagnosis of pregnancy.

II. Initial antepartum assessment

A. Purpose of initial antepartum visit[1,22]
   1. Introduce woman to provider and to the health care system.
   2. Initiate the system of physician consultation and referral.

3. Initiate the system of nutritional, psychosocial, and health educational support.
4. Gather initial physical data base regarding woman and her family.
5. Gather initial psychosocial data base regarding woman and her family.
6. Gather initial laboratory value data base regarding woman, consistent with her gestational age.

B. History
 1. Demographic characteristics (e.g., age, race, marital status, socioeconomic status, and educational level)
 2. Medical and surgical history
 3. Family history
 4. Occupational exposures and allergies
 5. Previous obstetrical history
   a. Number of previous pregnancies
   b. Progress of previous pregnancies
   c. Outcome of previous pregnancies
     • Abortion: spontaneous or therapeutic
     • Antepartum complications
     • Preterm birth
     • Multiple gestation
     • Onset of labor: spontaneous or induced
     • Length of labor
     • Complications of labor
     • Setting for delivery (home, birthing center, hospital)
     • Type of delivery (forceps, vacuum, spontaneous, cesarean section [C section])
     • If C-section, type of uterine incision
     • Presentations and positions at birth
     • Analgesia and anesthesia
     • Condition of the perineum (episiotomy, lacerations)
     • Infant outcome: weight, Apgar, complications, current status
     • Postpartum course
 6. Current obstetrical history
   a. Contraceptive use prior to this gestation
   b. First day of LNMP and menstrual history
   c. Signs and symptoms of pregnancy to date
   d. Bleeding since LNMP
   e. Previous pregnancy test performed (when? where? type? results?)

C. Physical exam
 1. Physical assessment is conducted according to the procedure described in Chapter 1, with documentation of all changes consistent with the gestational age of the pregnancy.[5,25,27,48]
   a. Temperature tends to high normal values (96.4°-99.2°F) in first half of pregnancy.
   b. Pulse may increase 10-15 beats per minute.

    c. Respiratory rate increases up to 15 percent of normal.

    d. Blood pressure in the mid-trimester may dip slightly.

    e. Skin may increase in pigmentation (chloasma on face) and perspiration, linea nigra and striae may occur on abdomen or breasts.

    f. Nasal vasculature increases in friability.

    g. Mouth and/or gums may experience hyperplasia, hyperemia, and gum softening.

    h. Thyroid may enlarge slightly.

    i. Pulmonary system is affected by elevation of diaphragm, with increased respiratory rate and effort.

    j. Breasts experience pigmentation of nipples and areola, appearance of Montgomery's tubercules (note presence or absence of colostrum and inversion or eversion of nipples).

    k. Cardiac exam may reveal soft systolic flow murmurs.

    l. Musculoskeletal changes include increased lordosis of the spine and increased mobility of pelvic joints.

    m. Abdominal exam should note presence or absence of diastasis.

    n. Pelvic exam[2,55]

      • Presumptive signs of pregnancy are the following:

        — Chadwick's sign: a bluish discoloration of vaginal wall and vestibule

        — Goodell's sign: softening of cervix and vagina with increased leukorrhea

        — Hegar's sign: compressability and softening of the lower uterine segment

        — McDonald's sign: softening of the junction between the uterus and the cervix.

      • Provide woman with the opportunity to visualize external genitalia and cervix in a mirror, if she desires.

2. Conduct these additional assessments on the pregnant woman:

    a. Assess for probable signs of pregnancy:

      • Ballottement of fetal parts after 16th week

      • Assessment of uterine contractility (begins as early as 10th week but increases in intensity near term [Braxton-Hicks])

      • Progressive abdominal and uterine enlargement

      • Positive pregnancy test

      • Auscultation of placental souffle

    b. Measure fundal height.

    c. Assess fetal position (Leopold maneuvers) after 28 weeks.

    d. Assess for positive signs of pregnancy:

      • Auscultation of fetal heart tones

        — By ultrasonic assessment if > 10 but < 18-20 weeks gestation

        — By fetoscope if > 18-20 weeks gestation

      • Palpation of fetal movement

• Ultrasonic imaging of fetus (as early as 6th week)
• Palpation of the fetal outline (20 or more weeks of pregnancy)
D. Laboratory studies
   1. Routine assessments (Table 5-1)
      a. Blood type and Rh factor[6,33]
        • Obtain at initial visit.
        • If Rh negative, investigate father's Rh status.
      b. Antibody screen and identification
        • Obtain at initial visit on all women.
        • Obtain at 26 weeks for mothers anticipating antepartum Rh immune prophylaxis or at 28 and 36 weeks for Rh-unsensitized mothers not receiving Rh immune prophylaxis.
        • Obtain additional screens for mothers with other positive antibodies that can cause hemolytic disease (anti-Kell is the most common of unusual antibodies).
      c. Hemoglobin or hematocrit (complete blood count)
        • Obtain at initial visit on all women.
        • Repeat at 32 weeks on selected women.
        • Repeat sooner to assess efficacy of therapy for anemia as appropriate.
      d. Gonorrhea culture
        • Screen all women at initial visit.
        • Repeat as indicated, especially following possible exposure.
      e. Pap smear
        • Obtain at initial visit on all women unless done recently.
        • Repeat as indicated, e.g., as follow-up for abnormal findings.
      f. Rubella titer
        • Screen all women at initial visit.
        • Obtain serial titers to diagnose infection if nonimmune mother is exposed during pregnancy.
      g. Urinalysis or urine culture and sensitivity
        • Screen all women at initial visit.
        • Repeat as indicated for diagnosis of women experiencing signs and symptoms of urinary tract infection (UTI).
        • Repeat in second and third trimester for women who have a history of frequent UTIs and/or pyelonephritis in previous pregnancies.
      h. VDRL-FTA (Veneral Disease Research Laboratory—Flourescent Trepomema Antibody)
        • Screen all women at initial visit.
        • Repeat if exposure is suspected.
   2. Selected assessments
      a. Alpha fetoprotein in maternal serum[33,35]
        • Obtain at 15-18 weeks for the following women:
          — Those with a history of infant with neural tube defect
          — Those with a strong family history of neural tube defect

TABLE 5.1
Lab Value Changes in Pregnancy

Test	Change in Pregnancy	Prepregnancy Value	Pregnancy Value
Blood			
Hgb*	None	12-15	
Hct†	↓; peak at 28 wks	37-47	> 34
WBC‡	↑	4500 cell/mm^3	7500-9000 cell/mm^3 (14,000-15,000 not unusual)
Platlets	↑ by one third	150-350,000	> 200,000
Fibrinogen	↑ by 50%	350 (250-400)	500
Retic § count	↑	0.5-1.5	
Coagubility	↓	12 min	8 min
Lipids	↑	650	1000
Cholesterol	↑	180	260
Fasting blood sugar	↓	70-115	< 100
BUN$^#$	↓	10-15	< 5
Creatinine	↓		< 0.6
Uric acid	↓	3-7.5	< 5
Na$^+$	None		
K$^+$	None		
Cl$^+$	None		
Urine (24 hours)			
Protein	↑	10-100 mg	< 300 mg
Cr¶ clearance	↑	105-132	150-225

* Hgb = hemoblobin
† Hct = hemotocrit
‡ WBC = white blood count
§ Retic = reticuloc
\# BUN = blood urea nitrogen
¶ Cr = creatinine

— Those from a geographically high-risk population
- Offer at 15-18 weeks to all women under guidelines effective in several states.

b. Genetic counseling for amniocentesis or chorionic villi sampling. Refer women before 20 weeks gestation (ideally as soon as pregnant), who may have one of the following:
- Family history of birth defects, or mental retardation
- Extended family history of known genetic disease, e.g., neuro-fibromatosis, hemophilia, cystic fibrosis.
- Obstetrical history of multiple miscarriages (> 3) or perinatal deaths
- Infant with congenital anomaly, birth defect, or mental retardation
- Inclusion in ethnic or racial groups at high risk for specific genetic diseases, such as sickle cell anemia, Tay-Sachs disease, and thalassemia.
- Age 35 or older.
- High risk factors, such as insulin-dependent diabetes, and ingestion of known teratogens (including alcohol)

c. G_6PD (glucose 6 dehydrogenase deficiency) assessment: done on women of black or Middle East descent especially if there is a history of severe anemia

d. Glucose screen[18,21]
- Obtain on initial visit for women with the following:
  — Obesity (> 170 pounds prepregnant weight or > 30 percent ideal body weight for height).
  — History of previous infant over 8½ pounds (3856 g)
  — History of gestational diabetes
  — Strong family history of diet- or insulin-dependent diabetes in parents, or siblings
  — History of previous fetal or neonatal death
  — Age greater than 35
- Screen all women at 24-28 weeks gestation.

e. Hepatitis B antigen (HBAg)
- Obtain on initial visit for women with history of the following:
  — IV drug use
  — Hepatitis B or exposure
  — Southeast Asian descent
  — Health employees exposed to contaminated blood products, e.g., dialysis and lab personnel.

f. Herpes type II culture
- Obtain a culture of lesion and/or cervix at initial visit for women with the following:
  — Vulvar or cervical lesions
  — Strong history of prior infection
  — Recent exposure
- Screen all women who have had a positive lesion during pregnancy at least once at 36 weeks or more of gestation

g. HIV virus (human immunodeficiency virus)
  • Screening or referral should be made for women in the following high-risk groups:
    — Known prostitutes
    — Known IV drug users
    — Spouses of HIV-antigen-positive people or people with AIDS or AIDS-related complex (ARC)
    — Patients with medical conditions requiring frequent blood transfusions and/or blood products
h. Renal function tests (BUN, creatinine, uric acid)
  • Obtain baseline screen for women with:
    — Hypertension
    — Renal disease
    — Hypertensive disorders of pregnancy
  • Repeat as indicated, e.g., in patients experiencing signs and symptoms of pregnancy induced hypertension (PIH).
i. Sickle cell trait-Hgb electrophoresis: screen Black and Middle Eastern women
j. Thyroid Panel (T3, T4, free thyroid index)
  • Screen at initial visit for women with the following:
    — History of or presently taking thyroid supplementation
    — Presence of enlarged thyroid
k. Tuberculin skin testing: screen women dependent on agency protocol, especially in high-risk geographical locales
E. Management
  1. Order appropriate laboratory tests.[54]
  2. Order vitamin and iron supplementations as appropriate.
  3. Arrange for consultation for identified problems.
  4. Arrange for referral to nutrition programs if appropriate and patient is eligible.
  5. Arrange for scheduled return visits.
F. Teaching for the normal exam
  1. Orient woman to system of prenatal care, setting, and provider.
  2. Discuss schedule of prenatal visits and anticipated laboratory tests.
  3. Provide nutritional goals and weight objectives.
  4. Discuss additional nutritional requirements and vitamin supplementation for pregnancy.
  5. Discuss expected developmental patterns for both mother and fetus.
  6. Inform woman of possible danger signs and symptoms of pregnancy problems as appropriate to current gestational age, with information on how to contact provider.

III. Continuing antepartum assessment

A. Purpose of the return visit
  1. Monitor the progress of the pregnancy along the following parameters:

      a. Fetal development

      b. Fetal well-being

      c. Maternal physiological adaptation

      d. Maternal psychosocial adaptation

  2. Monitor family adaptation to ongoing pregnancy.

  3. Promote nutritional well-being through review and counseling.

  4. Provide and discuss appropriate health education.

  5. Direct family in formulating a birth plan.

B. History

  1. Inquire about concerns, problems, or questions since last visit.

  2. Elicit presence of common complaints of pregnancy.

  3. Obtain interval medical history and/or visits to medical facility or practitioner.

  4. Assess compliance with ongoing therapies.

  5. Obtain nutritional status and diet history if indicated.

  6. Assess social situation (marital, sexual, educational, and occupational).

  7. Ask about perception of fetal movement.

C. Physical exam

  1. Assess urine for presence of glucose and protein.

  2. Assess blood pressure and pulse.

  3. Assess both total weight gain/loss and gain/loss since last visit.

  4. Measure fundal height and compare with expected growth based on estimated date of confinement (EDC).

  5. Conduct Leopold maneuvers to determine fetal lie and presentation.

  6. Auscultate the fetal heart tones.

  7. Assess degree of dependent edema; check reflexes if indicated.

D. Laboratory studies: as indicated (see Section II, D)

E. Management

  1. Order appropriate laboratory tests.

  2. Order initial or continuing medications as indicated by results of laboratory review.

  3. Initiate therapy for identified discomforts of pregnancy.

  4. Initiate or follow-up consultation for identified problems of pregnancy.

  5. Arrange for return prenatal visits.

    a. Recommended schedule of return visits

      • Once per month until the 28th week

      • Every 2 weeks from 28 to 36 weeks

      • Every week from 36 weeks to delivery.

    b. Additional visits are recommended:

      • At 20 weeks: to document presence of the fetal heart rate with use of fetoscope

      • Weekly from 24 to 36 weeks: to conduct cervical examination for patients who are at high risk for and/or symptomatic of premature labor

      • Twice weekly from 42 weeks gestation to delivery

F. Teaching for the normal exam
  1. Provide appropriate teaching for identified concerns or problems.
  2. Teach developmental growth and changes as appropriate to gestational age.[2,40]
  3. Provide anticipatory guidance for routine laboratory reassessments and schedule of return visits.
  4. Continue discussion of birth planning including birth options, e.g., anesthesia, circumcision, site of birth, and delivery positions.

IV. Management of common discomforts of pregnancy

A. **Backache**
  1. History
     a. Onset, location, and duration of symptoms
     b. Concurrent symptoms of UTI or onset of labor[1,2,18,22,30,31,41,46,47,52]
     c. Relationship of symptoms to occupational exposure or event, including household activities
     d. Symptoms of neurological impingement (e.g., herniated disc, sciatica) such as radiation to legs, sensory changes in legs, and sphincter difficulties
     e. Relief therapies already attempted and their efficacy
  2. Physical exam
     a. Assess degree of lordosis.
     b. Check for scoliosis.
     c. Assess for costovertebral angle tenderness.
     d. Rule out tumors or lesions developed since last exam.
     e. Conduct brief neurological (sensorimotor) exam of lower extremities.
     f. Rule out labor by cervical exam if indicated.
  3. Laboratory studies: Urinalysis or urine culture and sensitivity if urinary symptoms are present
  4. Differential diagnosis
     a. Prodromal or preterm labor contractions
     b. Deficit in lumbosacral vertebral column
     c. Urinary tract infection
  5. Management and teaching[30]
     a. Demonstrate proper posture and provide corrective exercises as appropriate.
     b. Instruct on proper body mechanics for lifting.
     c. Massage affected part.
     d. Apply heat or ice to local area.
     e. Recommend low-heeled shoes for walking and standing.
     f. Encourage side-lying with slightly bent knees for sleep (reduces lordosis).
     g. Instruct on pelvic tilt, back strengthening, and abdominal tightening exercises.
     h. Suggest a maternity girdle for women with poor abdominal tone, par-

ticularly gravid multiparas and obese clients.
   i. Provide nutritional guidance for the obese women.
   j. Prescribe non-aspirin analgesic PO every 4-6 hrs. PRN.
   k. Advise woman that physical causes of backache have obstetrical and anesthetic considerations, and refer as necessary.
B. **Constipation**
   1. History
      a. Frequency of fecal evacuation
      b. Increasing firmness and compactness of fecal material
      c. Bloating and associated abdominal discomfort
      d. Increased flatulence
      e. Symptoms of pica
      f. Diet and fluid intake
      g. Therapies already tried and their efficacy
      h. Iron supplementation: dosage and compliance
      i. Activity level
      j. Presence of blood in stool
      k. Narcotic use (methadone, codeine)
   2. Physical exam
      a. Palpate for generalized or localized abdominal pain.
      b. Auscultate bowel sounds for increase/decrease/absence.
      c. Palpate presence of firm stool in rectum.
      d. Identify hemorrhoids or tumors by inspection and digital exam.
   3. Laboratory studies: obtain stool for blood, ova, and parasites, if indicated by patient report of blood in stool
   4. Differential diagnosis: bowel obstruction, which presents ultimately as an acute abdominal emergency
   5. Management[30,56]
      a. Suggest natural laxatives such as prune juice or a fiber drink such as psyllium hydrophilic mucilloid (Metamucil, 1 teaspoon. QD to TID).
      b. Increase fluid intake to six to eight glasses of fluid daily.
      c. Increase fiber in diet (fruits, vegetables, and bran cereals).
      d. Increase exercise/activity level.
      e. Prescribe stool softener (not recommended for long-term use) as appropriate, e.g., docusate (Colace), 100 mg QD or BID PO.
      f. Use of enemas (Fleets, soap solution) may be necessary in extreme cases that have progressed to impaction, however, they are generally inadvisable due to their uterine stimulating effects.
      g. Refer for consultation and sigmoidoscopic examination for all abnormal findings.
   6. Teaching
      a. Encourage the establishment of regular bowel habits.
      b. The woman should be advised never to ignore the urge to defecate as retained stool loses fluid and compacts more firmly.
      c. Mineral oil should be avoided as a therapy since it prevents absorption

of fat soluble vitamins.
  d. Excessive reliance on laxatives can be habituating.
  e. Straining at stool can lead to hemorrhoid formation and vasovagal syn-
     cope.
  f. Several laxatives that can be purchased as over the counter therapies are
     extremely harsh and may cross the placenta affecting the baby. (Milk of
     Magnesia is the exception.) Inform woman to consult provider before
     ingesting.

C. Dyspnea
  1. History
     a. Onset and duration of symptoms
     b. Relationship of symptoms to exertion or position
     c. Woman's and family's history of asthma/allergies
     d. Woman's history of cardiac disease
     e. Smoking history
  2. Physical exam
     a. Observe for flaring of nostrils (extreme dyspnea).
     b. Auscultate lungs for ventilation, rales, rhonchi, and wheezing.
     c. Reassess cardiac exam.
     d. Evaluate fundal height in relation to diaphragm.
  3. Laboratory studies: none indicated
  4. Differential diagnosis
     a. Cardiovascular disease
     b. Pulmonary disease
     c. Asthma
     d. Respiratory allergies
  5. Management
     a. Attention to posture, both standing and sitting, may be of help in late
        pregnancy.
     b. Refer all cases of dyspnea accompanied by cardiac murmur or altered
        pulmonary breath sounds to physician for diagnosis and management.
  6. Teaching [30]
     a. Advise woman that smoking may aggravate dyspneic condition.
     b. Smaller more frequent meals will alleviate the compounding effect of
        stomach pressure on the diaphragm.
     c. Dyspnea can be *induced* by certain psychoprophylactic breathing exer-
        cises or postures. Woman must be cautioned to be alert for this
        phenomenon.[47]
     d. An extra pillow to elevate the head may also be helpful for sleep.
     e. Diaphragm lifting exercises (arms above head) may provide temporary
        relief.
     f. Self help strategies for structured, controlled breathing, such as those
        used by asthmatics, may be of some help during acute dyspneic
        episodes.

D. **Edema**
  1. History
     a. Onset of symptoms relative to
        • Time of day (present on waking or at end of day)
        • Activities (work, shopping, etc.)
     b. Association with dietary excesses (e.g., salt)
     c. Use of constricting garments (e.g., garters)
     d. Relief measures previously used and their efficacy
  2. Physical exam
     a. Observe puffiness of lower legs, ankles, feet, and face.
     b. Assess presence of pitting of skin when compressed by touch.
     c. Note aching and discomfort of lower extremities.
     d. Observe possible venous distention.
     e. Check blood pressure.
  3. Laboratory studies: urine dipstick for protein
  4. Differential diagnosis
     a. Hypertensive disorders of pregnancy
     b. Thrombophlebitis for leg edema
  5. Management and teaching
     a. Avoid prolonged standing or sitting.
     b. Avoid constrictive clothing such as knee-high hosiery or garters.
     c. Elevate feet during mid-day rest periods, slightly above the level of the heart.
     d. Instruct woman regarding the physiological benefits of the left side lying position for sleep or rest.
     e. Use of support hosiery may be helpful.
     f. If support hosiery is to be worn, it should be put on before arising.
     g. Increase fluid intake to increase renal perfusion and natural diuresis.
     h. Restriction of dietary sodium intake is no longer advisable. Extensive sodium restriction stimulates kidney reabsorption of the element.
     i. Chemical diuretics should also be avoided as they may result in depletion of salt and potassium reserves in both mother and baby.

E. **Epistaxis**
  1. History
     a. Occurrence of spontaneous nose bleeds in absence of trauma
     b. Persistent nasal stuffiness.
     c. Habit of vigorous nose blowing or nose picking
     d. Use of sniffed drugs such as inhalation of cocaine, glue
  2. Physical exam
     a. Assess blood pressure as normal for the stage of pregnancy.
     b. Inspect nasal system for ulceration, polyps, or trauma.
  3. Laboratory studies
     a. None indicated in general

b. Hematocrit determination useful following significant and multiple events
4. Differential diagnosis
   a. Ulceration of nasal membrane secondary to earlier trauma or cocaine abuse
   b. Epistaxis secondary to high blood pressure (200/120)
5. Management and teaching[48]
   a. Elevate head.
   b. Apply pressure to the bleeding nostril(s) for at least 15 minutes.
   c. Apply ice or cold cloths to selected areas: bridge of nose, back of neck.
   d. Instill normal saline nose drops PRN.
   e. Refer severe cases for electrocautery of nasal vessels.
   f. Provide nasal packing for severe bleeding.
   g. Caution woman to avoid vigorous nose blowing and nose picking.

F. Heartburn
1. History
   a. Relationship of symptoms to mealtimes and foods eaten
   b. Duration of symptoms
   c. Location and radiation of burning sensation, (along rib chest wall or concentrated in mid-sternal area)
   d. Associated burping
2. Physical exam: abdominal assessment
   a. Fundal height in relation to upper abdominal organs
   b. Normal size and contours of spleen, pancreas, and liver (assessment dependent on gestational age)
3. Laboratory studies: none indicated
4. Differential diagnosis
   a. Hiatal hernia
   b. Gastric ulcer
5. Management and teaching
   a. Encourage smaller, more frequent meals.
   b. Encourage avoidance of fried foods and fats in diet.
   c. Alert woman to posture while sitting and standing postingestion. Discourage lying down postingestion.
   d. Woman should elevate head 30° while sleeping.
   e. Milk is a basic coating agent for stomach.
   f. Suggest antacid preparation ingestion half hour prior to meals and at bedtime. Usual dose is 2 tablespoons. Concentrated (double) doses are available and more efficacious.[7]
      • Aluminum hydroxide $Al(OH)_3$: Gelusil or Amphojel
      • Calcium carbonate $Ca(CO)_3$: Tums
      • Magnesium hydroxide $Mg(OH)_3$: Maalox, Mylanta, or Riopan
      • Simethicone: Gaviscon
   g. Antacids containing sodium bicarbonate ($NaHCO_3$) should be avoided

as they decrease absorption of B-complex vitamins and promote fluid retention.

G. **Hemorrhoids**
   1. History
      a. Feeling of fullness in anal/rectal area
      b. Pain and itching associated with defecation
      c. Slight bleeding associated with defecation
      d. Presence of constipation
   2. Physical exam
      a. Observe for external hemorrhoid
      b. Palpate for internal hemorrhoid
   3. Laboratory studies
      a. Stool for ova and parasites may be indicated to rule out other causes of rectal bleeding.
      b. Hgb or Hct may be indicated.
   4. Differential diagnosis: thrombosis of rectal veins
   5. Management
      a. Prescribe stool-softening agents (docusate, 100 mg PO QD or BID).
      b. Suggest psyllium hydrophilic mucilloid (Metamucil), 1 teaspoon in 8 ounces of water one to three times a day.
      c. Order hemorrhoidal suppositories or creams; however, avoid those with hydrocortisone during pregnancy.
      d. Instruct woman to use warm sitz baths: 20 minutes three times a day.
      e. Apply witch hazel compresses to external hemorrhoids.
      f. Apply topical anesthetic ointments following each bowel movement.
      g. Encourage side-lying position with elevated hips.
      h. Apply ice bag or pack 30 minutes TID (to promote retraction).
      i. Reinsert the hemorrhoids in concert with perineal tightening exercises, if possible.
      j. Refer for ligation and excision as appropriate.
   6. Teaching
      a. Provide nutritional advice regarding fiber and fluid.
      b. Increased activity may be helpful to increase peristalsis.
      c. Regular bowel habits may help to reduce incidence of constipation, which aggravates hemorrhoidal symptoms.

H. **Insomnia**
   1. History
      a. Onset and duration of symptoms
      b. Association with bladder fullness, heartburn, dyspnea, or fetal activity
      c. Association with use of stimulants (caffeine, drugs)
      d. Social and emotional stress patterns
   2. Physical Exam: as appropriate to history of associated symptoms (section IV, H, 1,b)
   3. Laboratory studies: none indicated

4. Management and teaching
   a. Instruct in supportive comfort measures to reduce stress and promote sleep.
      • Suggest warm shower, bath, or massage prior to bedtime.
      • Instruct in stress reduction, e.g., conscious relaxation techniques.
      • Suggest warm milk or fluids before bedtime.
      • Discuss more comfortable sleeping positions.
   b. Engage in mild to moderate exercise, e.g., walking, during the day.
   c. Woman should avoid alcohol, caffeine, and other stimulants.
   d. Barbiturate sleeping pills in second and third trimester should be used with great discretion and physician consultation.

I. **Leg cramps**
   1. History
      a. Frequency and duration of spontaneous cramping spasms of calves or thighs
      b. Relationship of symptoms to activity level
      c. Dietary intake of calcium and phosphorus
   2. Physical exam
      a. Elicit Homan's sign: negative response desired.
      b. Inspect for redness and heat in extremities.
   3. Laboratory studies: if discomfort persists
      a. Serum calcium level
      b. Serum phosphorus level
   4. Differential diagnosis: thrombophlebitis
   5. Management[52]
      a. Recommend altered diet to reduce phosphorus and increase calcium intake (although this cause-management combination is not reported in recent literature)—e.g., calcium lactate, 0.6 g PO TID with meals (particularly in lactose-intolerant clients).
      b. Recommend aluminum hydroxide liquid, 1 g PO TID before meals.
   6. Teaching
      a. Calcium lactate increases amount of ionized calcium in the plasma.
      b. Aluminum hydroxide gel binds phosphorus in the intestinal tract and prevents absorption.
      c. Kneading or rubbing the affected muscle may provide symptomatic relief but should not be done if pain is persistent, which could indicate phlebitis.
      d. Dorsiflexion of the food extends the contracted muscle and provides counter relief.

J. **Nausea and vomiting**
   1. History
      a. Onset of symptoms: time of day and gestational age
      b. Frequency of symptoms
      c. How much food and fluid is retained

d. Presence of blood in vomitus
e. Associated salivation
f. Relationship of symptoms to food/fluid/supplements ingested
2. Physical exam
a. Evaluate for pallor and paleness of skin.
b. Note loss of skin turgor secondary to dehydration.
c. Palpate abdomen for pain, masses, and pregnancy assessment.
d. Assess vital signs.
e. Note weight change: gain or loss.
3. Laboratory studies: urine for ketones, if large ketones are present, obtain serum acetone
4. Differential diagnosis
a. Gastrointestinal disturbances
b. Bacterial or viral influenzas
c. Psychogenic disturbances
d. Molar pregnancy
e. Hyperemesis of pregnancy
5. Management and teaching
a. Ingest dry crackers or bread before arising in morning and at first symptoms of nausea.
b. Decrease fluid intake, especially with meals.
c. Eat smaller, more frequent meals.
d. Avoid fatty and spicy foods and offensive odors.
e. Sit upright after meals.
f. Increase ingestion of vitamin B (milk, meat, fish, poultry, eggs, whole or enriched grain cereals, breads and flours).
g. Suggest vitamin B_6, 50 mg PO TID. If necessary, increase to total of six doses per day, then decrease gradually.
h. Take doxylamine, 10 mg PO, two at hour of sleep (h.s.), one in morning, with one additional in afternoon, if needed.
i. Take Emetrol (fructose, glucose, and orthophosphoric acid), 1-2 tablespoons PO, upon arising. Repeat every 3 hours or whenever nausea threatens.
j. Obtain physician consult for other antiemetic agents, if above therapies are ineffective.
k. Refer for possible IV vitamins or fluid supplementation for weight loss of over 5 pounds, or inability to retain food for over 24 hours, or if serum ketones are present.
l. Refer patient for psychosocial assessment or support as indicated by patient's situation.
K. **Pica**
1. History
a. Craving and eating of substances that may or may not be foods, e.g., clay, laundry and corn starch, plastic, soap, toothpaste, and ice.

        b. Exclusion of other nutritional foods and supplements.
    2. Physical exam
        a. Note pallor of skin and mucous membranes (anemia).
        b. Observe for jaundice (local ingestion or toxicity).
    3. Laboratory studies
        a. Draw hemoglobin or hematocrit to determine if pica is leading to anemia.
        b. Obtain additional studies as appropriate to the craved substance, e.g., serum lead levels if painted plaster is ingested.
    4. Management
        a. Order or perform nutritional assessment and counseling.
        b. Provide nutritional supplementation as appropriate.
    5. Teaching
        a. Counsel as appropriate to the substance craved; woman must be advised regarding the nature of selected substances and their potential harmful effects.

L. **Round ligament pain**
    1. History
        a. Presence of sharp intermittent discomfort localized to the lower quadrants of the abdomen and to the inguinal area
        b. Relationship of symptoms to sudden change in posture
c. Absence of associated fever or other abdominal discomfort
    2. Physical exam
        a. Palpate for masses and tenderness in inguinal area.
        b. Palpate the round ligament itself to reproduce symptoms (thin women only).
        c. Evaluate need for further pelvic assessment to rule out pelvic infectious disease (unlikely in absence of associated symptoms).
        d. Conduct passive or active leg lifts from the supine position. (Associated discomfort in the inguinal area is almost always diagnostic).
    3. Laboratory studies: none indicated
    4. Differential diagnosis
        a. Appendicitis
        b. Constipation
        c. Ectopic pregnancy
        d. Gallbladder disease
        e. Separation of symphysis pubis
        f. Pelvic thrombophlebitis
    5. Management
        a. Suggest warm baths for relief.
        b. Apply heating pad to local area.
        c. Sauna and whirlpool baths have been suggested; however, temperatures above 110° F should not be sustained for over 10 minutes, to avoid an effect on the body core temperature.[36]

    d. Differentiate between intermittent pain as a single symptom and pain associated with fever and other abdominal discomfort.

    e. Consult or refer for prolonged pain, radiating pain, and pain associated with severe nausea and vomiting, diarrhea, or bleeding.

6. Teaching

    a. Avoid sudden changes in posture and position, particularly side-to-side motion.

    b. Maternity girdles may be of some comfort, especially if poor abdominal tone exists.

M. Varicosities

1. History

    a. Onset of symptoms of dull aching extremities

    b. Associated edema

    c. History of varicosities in family

    d. Association with prolonged standing or sitting, e.g., in occupational setting

2. Physical exam

    a. Weigh patient.

    b. Elicit negative Homan's sign.

    c. Note appearance of network of blue or purple rope-like veins on surface of affected body part.

    d. Note edema for severity and location.

3. Laboratory studies: none indicated

4. Differential diagnosis

    a. Spider angioma

    b. Phlebitis

5. Management and teaching

    a. Exercise in moderation promotes fluid return from extremities.

    b. Rest, several times per day, with legs elevated to 30°; however, caution against elevation of the legs to a degree that requires patient to be flat on her back, in order to avoid supine hypotension syndrome.

    c. Use support panty hosiery while standing and walking. Support hosiery, to be most effective, should be put on before arising from bed.

    d. Avoid garters and similar constrictive articles of clothing.

    e. Avoid excessive standing, sitting, or crossing of the legs. (Inquire about employment requirements.)

    f. Vulvar varicosities may be supported by firm application of a perineal pad.

    g. Increase fluids to discourage concentrated (sluggish) venous return.

    h. Begin birth planning for alternative delivery positions.

    i. Refer for Doppler evaluation of the blood flow and for physician consultation and management should signs of phlebitis occur.

    j. Ligation and stripping of the veins may be done after pregnancy in severe cases.

k. Provide prescriptive hosiery (Teds, Jobst) as severity warrants.

V. Management of deviations from normal in the antepartum period

A. **Iron-deficiency anemia**[41]
   1. History
      a. Previous anemia: pregnant and nonpregnant
      b. Compliance with supplemental and nutritional therapies
      c. Fatigue, weakness, and malaise
      d. Apathy and lassitude
      e. Headache
   2. Physical exam
      a. Take pulse: tachycardia may be present if anemic.
      b. Obtain respiratory rate: dypsnea may be indicative of anemia.
      c. Assess for edema.
      d. Assess for pallor and pale mucous membranes.
   3. Laboratory studies
      a. Obtain initial CBC with red cell indices.
      b. Supplemental tests may be helpful:
         • Platelet count (will be normal or increased)
         • Reticulocyte count (will be normal or increased)
      c. Consult physician following receipt of the following diagnostic tests (usually done after unsuccessful 4-week trial of iron supplementation). Suspect iron deficiency anemia if any of the following are true:
         • Total iron binding capacity is elevated.
         • Serum iron level is below 50-60 µg/100 ml
         • Saturation (serum iron/total iron binding capacity) is less than 10 percent.
         • Blood smear shows microcytic, hypochromic RBCs.
      d. Obtain the following to assist with differential diagnosis:
         • Sickle cell prep and/or Hgb electrophoresis
         • Serum folate levels, which may be decreased with folic acid deficiency
         • G_6PD
         • Stool for guiac, ova, and parasites
   4. Differential diagnosis
      a. Acquired anemias
         • Posthemorrhagic
         • Folic acid deficiency (megaloblastic)
         • Hemolytic (secondary to drugs such as sulfonamide, aspirin, nitrofurans and quinine)
         • Hemolytic (transfusion reaction)
         • Pernicious (vitamin B_{12} deficiency)
      b. Inherited anemias include:
         • Sickle cell

- Sickle cell hemoglobin C disease
- Thalassemia
- Congenital hemolytic
- Glucose 6 Phosphate Dehydrogenase deficiency
5. Management and teaching
   a. Provide nutritional management
      - Recommend iron-rich foods (liver, lean meats, legumes, fish, egg yolk, enriched breads and cereals, whole grains, dark leafy vegetables, molasses, and dried fruits).
      - Vitamin C helps to increase absorption of iron from the GI tract; supplements should be taken with citrus juice or with citrus fruits.
      - Milk, calcium carbonate, and tea interfere with iron absorption.
   b. Recommend dietary supplementation
      - Woman should intake up to 200 mg of elemental iron per day, by mouth:
        — Ferrous fumarate, 600 mg (supplied as 300-mg sustained-release tablets)
        — Ferrous gluconate, 1660 mg (supplied as 225-mg tablets)
        — Ferrous sulfate, 1000 mg (supplied as 325-mg tablets)
      - Ingestion of iron on an empty stomach increases intestinal absorption.
      - Ingestion of iron at bedtime may help to reduce the incidence of nausea
      - Time-released iron capsules may be prescribed if tablet iron causes extreme nausea.
      - Iron will cause stools to turn black and may cause constipation.
   c. Consult for anemia of pregnancy unresponsive to dietary alteration. Hematocrit levels below 30 mgm % or Hgb less than 10 g requires assessment and definitive medical management.
   d. Repeat Hct and Hgb measurement 4 weeks following initiation of supplemental therapy.
   e. Parenteral injection of iron may be used in rare and serious deficiencies-only after physician consultation.
B. **Excessive weight gain**
   1. History
      a. Increase in excess of 2 pounds per week in the last trimester of pregnancy, or any increase in excess of 35 pounds over prepregnant weight.[56]
      b. Associated symptoms of decreased urine output
      c. Diet history: amount, frequency, and types of food eaten in interval since last visit (in particular, during previous 3 days).
   2. Physical exam
      a. Note presence or absence of edema.
      b. Note blood pressure and rule out PIH.
      c. Note respiratory and pulse rates to rule out concurrent cardiovascular events.

      d. Assess fundal height for rate of fetal growth.

  3. Laboratory studies

      a. If fundal height is inappropriately excessive, order sonogram to rule out multiple gestation and hydramnios.

      b. Order glucose screening.

  4. Differential diagnosis

      a. Hypertensive disorder of pregnancy with edema

      b. Multiple gestation

      c. Hydramnios

      d. Maternal diabetes with macrosomic fetus

  5. Management and teaching

      a. Provide nutritional counseling for controlled weight gain.

        • Weight loss in pregnancy is undesirable.

        • Controlled weight gain emphasizing protein and calorie counting is ideal weight management protocol.

      b. Weight gain in association with other clinical features suggestive of other complications (see above) should be assessed by laboratory studies and referred for consultation and management.

      c. Encourage moderate exercise.

C. Inadequate weight gain

  1. History

      a. Document total weight gain in pregnancy of less than 10 kg (22 pounds) and/or less than 1.0 kg each month during the last two trimesters.[42,56]

      b. Determine presence of nausea and vomiting.

      c. Ask about fatigue and anemia.

      d. Determine association with hyperactive metabolic state (pulse, respiration, and perspiration).

      e. Obtain diet history for intolerance for selected foods or fluids.

      f. Determine presence of social and environmental stressors.

  2. Physical exam

      a. Observe vital signs.

      b. Observe for skin pallor or turgor.

  3. Laboratory studies

      a. Obtain hemoglobin or hematocrit.

      b. Measure serum iron and folate levels as appropriate.

  4. Differential diagnosis

      a. Anorexia nervosa or bulimia

      b. Hypermetabolic body states or conditions

      c. Malabsorption syndrome

  5. Management

      a. Provide nutritional counseling for controlled weight gain.

      b. Supplement diet with selected vitamin and mineral elements—in particular, iron, calcium, and folic acid—to current recommended levels (see Table 5-2).

TABLE 5.2
Recommended Daily Dietary Allowances for Women (Revised 1980) From the Food and Nutrition Board of the National Academy of Sciences/National Research Council

Age (yr)	Weight (lb)	Height (in.)	Protein (g)	Fat-Soluble Vitamins			Water-Soluble Vitamins							Minerals					
				Vita-min A (µg)	Vita-min D (µg)	Vita-min E (mg)	Vita-min C (mg)	Thia-mine (mg)	Ribo-flavin (mg)	Niacin (mg)	Vita-min B (mg)	Folacin (µg)	Vita-min B (µg)	Calcium (mg)	Phos-phorus (mg)	Magne-sium (mg)	Iron (mg)	Zinc (mg)	Iodine (µg)
11-14	101	62	46	800	10	8	50	1.1	1.3	15	1.8	400	3.0	1200	1200	300	18	15	150
15-18	120	64	46	800	10	8	60	1.1	1.3	14	2.0	400	3.0	1200	1200	300	18	15	150
19-22	120	64	44	800	7.5	8	60	1.1	1.3	14	2.0	400	3.0	800	800	300	18	15	150
23-50	120	64	44	800	5	8	60	1.0	1.2	13	2.0	400	3.0	800	800	300	18	15	150
Pregnant			+30	+200	+5	+2	+20	+0.4	+0.3	+2	+0.6	+400	+1.0	+400	+400	+150	*	+5	+25
Lactating			+20	+400	+5	+3	+40	+0.5	+0.5	+5	+0.5	+100	+1.0	+400	+400	+150	*	+10	+50

*The increased requirement during pregnancy cannot be met by the iron content of typical American diets nor by the existing iron stores of many women; therefore, the use of 30-60 mg of supplemental iron is recommended. Iron needs during lactation are not substantially different from those of nonpregnant women, but continued supplementation for mothers for 2-3 months after parturition is advisable to replenish stores depleted by pregnancy.

      c. Follow infant with serial ultrasonographic studies to rule out intra-uterine growth retardation and/or to predict if infant will be born small for gestational age.

      d. Woman may be followed at shorter prenatal intervals in order to monitor weight gain or loss.

      e. Severe cases, in particular those due to psychological or socio-emotional causes (e.g., anorexia) may need nutritional supplementation in the form of prepared feeding formulas under physician management.

   6. Teaching

      a. Insufficient weight gain with associated protein and caloric depletion can affect brain development of fetus.

      b. Megadoses (more than 10 times RDA) of several vitamins (A, D, E, and K) may be associated with fetal defects.

      c. Calcium supplements derived from bone meal and dolomite should be avoided, as they may contain lead, which is harmful to both mother and fetus.

D. **Gestational diabetes (carbohydrate intolerence, class A)**[20,23,37,49]

   1. History

      a. Excessive hunger

      b. Excessive urination

      c. Excessive thirst

      d. Rapid weight gain

      e. Family history of diabetes

      f. Previous obstetrical history of large-for-gestational-age infant, adverse pregnancy outcome, or gestational diabetes.

   2. Physical exam: note rapid growth of fundal height in relation to gestational age.

   3. Laboratory studies

      a. Sample urine for glucose 1 plus or more (glycosuria).

      b. Order 1-hour glucose screen following a 50-gm oral glucose load. A serum glucose value > 140 mg/dl is abnormal.

      c. If 1-hour screen is abnormal, order 3-hour glucose test following 100 g oral glucose load (Table 5-3). Two abnormal values are diagnostic for gestational diabetes.

   4. Differential diagnosis

      a. Lowered renal glucose threshhold (glycosuria without glycosemia)

      b. Diabetes mellitus, greater than Class A

   5. Management

Institutional policy will vary. Some settings may require that all women diagnosed as gestationally diabetic be followed by physicians or in special gestational diabetic clinics. Other settings may incorporate outpatient nurse-clinician or nurse-midwife and physician comanagement. In either case, the therapies indicated below are appropriate. Physician consultation and/or referral is always indicated once an abnormal glucose tolerance is identified.

Table 5-3
Three Hour Glucose Tolerence Test

Time of Sample	Upper Normal Serum Value (mg/dl)	Upper Normal Whole Blood (Dextrometer)
Fasting	105	90
One hour	190	165
Two hours	165	145
Three hours	145	125

Data are according to ACOG standard.
Data from Gabbe.[20]

   a. Glycosuria only
- Screen with 50-g glucose test.
- Two-hour postprandial glucose levels (value not to exceed 120 mg/dL) may be of value to follow patients who "pass" the 1-hour screening test but continue to have glucosuria.

   b. Gestational diabetes (glycosuria and glycosemia)[20,23,28]
- Order 2000-2400 KCal American Diabetic Association (ADA) diabetic diet (high fiber; CHO, 50 percent; protein, 20 percent; fat, 30 percent).
- Two-hour postprandial blood sugars should be performed every 2 weeks to 36 weeks and then weekly to delivery. Values must not exceed 120 mg/dl serum.
- Monitor maternal status biweekly or weekly. Therapeutic compliance is assessed by nutritional review, serum glucose assessment, and urinary glucose testing.
- Monitor fetal status by serial sonography for macrosomia and biophysical profile, at appropriate intervals as requested by examiner.
- Start weekly nonstress testing for assessment of fetal well-being at 37 weeks.
- Conduct cervical assessment to determine readiness for induction and/or delivery weekly from 37 weeks.
- Deliver before 41 weeks gestation.

6. Teaching
   a. Procedures for administration of the glucose screening diagnostic tests will differ among institutions. Instruct patients regarding appropriate fasting or food and fluid intake for the appropriate glucose test to be effective and valid.
   b. Stress importance of proper calculation and utilization of the diabetic diet to control glycosemia.
   c. Instruct woman to monitor fetal activity with a fetal movement chart beginning at 34 weeks (Appendix A).
   d. Encourage moderate exercise. The effects of exercise as a therapeutic

adjunct to glucose control are being investigated, and current evidence seems to support such a program.

  e. Instruct woman that gestational diabetes indicates that the woman is "prediabetic." Her glucose tolerance curve may return to normal after delivery, but she is subject to return of the prediabetic state should subsequent stress occur. Moreover, she is predisposed to the development of diabetes. Emphasize importance of 6 week postpartum diabetic assessment.

E. **Intestinal Parasites**
  1. History
    a. Recent travel to endemic areas (Southeast Asia, Africa, Middle East, and parts of Central America)
    b. Recent migration from endemic areas
    c. Presence of constipation or diarrhea
    d. Presence of blood in stools (hookworm)
    e. Presence of anal-rectal itching (most parasites)
    f. Restlessness and irritable sleep (pinworms)
    g. Weight loss and fatigue (variable)
    h. Presence of these symptoms in family members
  2. Physical exam: inspect/palpate anus/rectum to rule out hemorrhoids/tumors as source of blood in stool
  3. Laboratory studies
    a. Stool specimen for identification of ova and cysts; three specimens collected sequentially are usually indicated
    b. Stool specimen for occult blood
    c. Hematocrit
  4. Differential diagnosis: loose diarrheal stools are more likely to contain life cycle stages of amoebas and flagellates than parasites
  5. Management[15] (treatment is listed in order of preferred regimens)

General principles
1. *Always treat malaria in pregnancy.*
2. *If **Entamoeba** is present, treat as an invasive pathogen.*
3. *Treat other parasites if patient is symptomatic, i.e., has severe anemia, diarrhea, or intestinal obstruction or is immunocompromised.*
4. *Patients who are not treated in pregnancy should be treated following childbirth, with appropriate consideration for breast- or bottle-feeding status.*

---

    a. Malaria
      • Always treat, including during pregnancy.
      • Obtain malaria prep.
      • Consult with physician if positive.
    b. *Entamoeba histolytica* (amebiasis)
      • Always treat, including during pregnancy, invasive-type pathogen because of complications of intestinal obstruction and worm migration.

Send specimen to microbiology lab to determine if it is of the invasive type (isoenzyme profile).
- Treat with one of the following:
  — Metronidazole (Flagyl), 250 mg PO BID x 10 days
  — Mebendazole (Vermox), 100 mg PO BID x 3 days (contraindicated during pregnancy, but okay with breast-feeding)
  — Pyrantel pamoate (Antiminth): single dose of 11 mg/1 kg to maximum dose of 1 g (probably safe during breast-feeding but has not been studied)
- Follow-up with stool for ova and parasites x 3 after treatment.
c. *Strongyloides stercoralis*
  - Treat if symptomatic.
  - Prescribe thiabendazole (Mintezol), 25 mg/kg PO BID x 2 days; (adults-children): x 5 days for disseminated strongyloides. Breast-feeding is contraindicated.
  - Follow-up with stool for ova and parasites x 3 after treatment.
d. *Ascaris lumbricoides* (roundworm)
  - Treat if symptomatic.
  - Treat with either:
    — Mebendazole (Vermox) 100 mg PO BID x 3 days (adults and children). May repeat after 3 weeks if not cured. Woman may breast-feed.
    — Pyrantel pamoate (Antiminth)—single dose of 11 mg/1 kg to maximum dose of 1 gm. Probably safe during breast-feeding.
e. *Taenia saginata* (tapeworm)
  - Always treat, except during pregnancy.
  - Treat with either:
    — Niclocide 2 g x 1-5 days, obtained from the Center for Disease Control (phone number: [404] 633-3311) or
    — Praziquantel, 10 mg/kg single dose
f. Hookworm
  - Treat only if anemia or significant gastrointestinal symptoms are present, or in children who lag behind on growth charts.
  - Mebendazole (Vermox) 100 mg PO BID x 3 days (adults and children over 2 years). Woman may breast-feed.
g. *Giardia lamblia*
  - Treat if symptomatic or low on growth chart.
  - Metronidazole (Flagyl) 250 mg PO TID x 10 days (pediatric dose 5 mg/kg). Woman should not breast-feed, although this is not well studied.
h. *Trichuris trichiura* (whipworm)
  - Treat if symptomatic or low on growth chart.
  - Mebendazole 100 mg PO BID x 3 days (adults and children over 2 years). Woman may breast-feed. May repeat after 3 weeks if not cured.

      i. *Enterobius vermicularis* (Pinworm)
- Treat only if symptomatic and not during pregnancy.
- Treat entire family simultaneously and repeat in 2 weeks.
- Treat with one of the following:
  — Pyrantel pamoate (Antiminth), 11 mg/kg x 1 dose
  — Mebendazole (Vermox), 100 mg x 1 dose. Woman may breast-feed.

7. Teaching
   a. Refrigerate stool specimens after collection unless directed otherwise.
   b. No food and diet restrictions are indicated before collection of the specimen.
   c. Avoid oily cathartics, e.g., mineral oil, as an aid to collection of the specimen as oil can obscure the microscopic examination.
   d. Maintain good personal hygiene in collection of the specimen to avoid reinfestation.
   e. Discuss importance of treatment of family members to cure their infestation and to prevent reinfestation, as appropriate.

F. **Hepatitis B antigen (positive)**
1. History
   a. Exposure to infected patients or previous disease history
   b. IV drug use
   c. Prostitution
   d. Work exposure to blood products and parenteral fluids
   e. Symptoms of disease are:
      - Malaise and lethargy
      - Light colored stools
      - Dark urine
      - Anorexia
      - Nausea, vomiting, and/or diarrhea
2. Physical exam: look for symptoms of disease state:
   a. Icterus of the skin
   b. Enlarged tender liver
   c. Mild splenomegaly
3. Laboratory studies
   a. Obtain serum for hepatitis B surface antigen (HBsAg) titers. Two positive titers taken at 6-month intervals indicate a positive carrier state in a newly exposed individual.[13]
   b. Additional serological markers that appear at various times are helpful in staging the course of the disease (Table 5-4).
   c. SGOT and SGPT are elevated during acute phase; this helps to differentiate the acute from the chronic carrier state.
4. Differential diagnosis: the demonstration of hepatitis antibody is diagnostic; additional causes of the symptoms cited for the hepatic disease include the following:
   a. Drug reactions

Table 5-4
Hepatitis B Virus (HBV) Markers

HBs*Ag	Anti-HBc†	Anti-HBs	Interpretation
-	-	-	No current or past hepatitis B virus (HBV) infection
+	-	-	New HBV infection before onset of symptoms
+	+	-	HBV infection: either new or chronic carrier
-	+	-	Either recently resolved HBV infection (before anti-HBs develops) or HBV carrier (HBsAg level too low to detect)
-	+	+	Past HBV infection; may be seen as early as 2-4 weeks after loss of HBsAg
-	-	+	Possible interpretations: (1) past HBV infection with loss of anti-HBc; (2) vaccine-induced antibody response; (3) nonspecific

*HBs = hepatitis B surface
†HBc = hepatitis B core

Data from Boehme[9]

    b. Pyelonephritis
    c. Cholestasis of pregnancy
    d. Pregnancy induced hypertension
    e. Gallstones
    f. Cirrhosis
    g. Fatty liver of pregnancy
  5. Management

The medical management of acute hepatitis is a physician responsibility. Practitioner management is directed toward prevention of disease transmission.

---

    a. Screen appropriate women prenatally to detect the hepatitis carrier.
    b. Identify carriers to protect the infant at birth by administration of HBIG (hepatitis B immune globulin). (The management of passive and active immunization of infants at birth is the responsibility of the pediatrician and well-baby care team.)
    c. Provide protection of the infant and health personnel by preventing exposure to all maternal blood and body fluids.
    d. Repeat antigen identification is required in all subsequent pregnancies to identify changes in the staging of hepatitis infective disease.
    e. Encourage hepatitis B vaccination postpartum for all mothers who have tested negative for HBsAg, but are at risk.
  6. Teaching

    a. Instruct woman that the incubation period for the onset of disease ranges from 30 to 180 days. Infants of carrier mothers are at particularly high risk. The transmission rate in first and second trimester is around 10 percent rising to 65 percent by the third trimester.

    b. Discuss with woman that hepatitis B surface antigen can be found in breast milk; however, breast-feeding is not contraindicated for infants who have received immunization.

G. **Herpes virus: genital (type I or II)**[34]

  1. History

    a. Primary infection
- Numerous vesicular lesions on all vaginal, anal, and cervical mucous membranes and perineal skin areas
- Low grade fever
- Pain, itching, burning, and tenderness of vesicles during healing process

    b. Secondary infection
- Symptoms as listed for the primary infection, but usually of lesser duration and intensity

  2. Physical exam

    a. Scrupulously examine perineum, vagina, and cervix for presence of lesions.

  3. Laboratory studies

    a. Obtain viral material for cytological studies (Tzanck smear) for giant cell changes in the cell nucleus (50 percent specific).

    b. Obtain culture for virologic studies of exudate (Hanks media).

  4. Differential diagnosis: primary chancre of syphilis

  5. Management[14,48]

    a. Suggest palliative treatment and support, including the following:
- Application of ice pack to area.
- Keeping area dry
- Urinating in warm water for symptomatic relief

    b. Document a positive herpes culture of any lesion noted during course of pregnancy.

    c. Perform at least one herpes viral culture at 36-37 weeks for all women with a positive culture in pregnancy or documented history of genital herpes virus.

    d. Pharmacologic therapy is available only for the nonpregnant woman (see Chapter 2).

    e. Refer all women with documented positive viral culture at or after 36 weeks of gestation, and all women with active lesions at the time of labor for physician management. Cesarean delivery may be indicated.

  6. Teaching

    a. Instruct woman that active herpetic lesions at time of delivery can be fatal to the infant who is infected, and document counseling.

    b. Stress to woman importance of reporting all symptoms suggestive of primary or recurrent disease.

    c. Discuss with woman that she is highly infective to others when lesions are present and must maintain strict pelvic isolation during that time.

H. **Pregnancy induced hypertension (PIH)**

  1. History

    a. General fatigue

    b. Headache

    c. Blurred and spotted vision

    d. Upper epigastric pain

    e. Nausea and vomiting

  2. Physical exam

    a. Elevated blood pressure (BP)

      • BP greater than or equal to 140/90 mm Hg on left side

      • Rise in systolic 30 mm Hg above baseline

      • Rise in diastolic 15 mm Hg above baseline

    b. Sudden weight gain of more than 2 pounds/each week documented

    c. Edema, particularly of face and hands

    d. Ankle clonus

    e. Proteinuria of 1 + or greater present

  3. Laboratory studies

    a. Baseline measures

      • Blood urea nitrogen

      • Creatinine

      • Uric acid

      • Platelets

      • Complete blood count

      • SGOT

    b. Diagnostic measures to follow:

      • Twenty-four-hour total urine protein

      • Twenty-four-hour urine creatinine clearance

  4. Differential diagnosis

    a. Essential (chronic) hypertension must be ruled out or acknowledged as a concurrent event.

    b. Dependent edema and excessive weight gain may be independent or concurrent events.

  5. Management[14,41]

    a. Prescribe bed rest, preferably on the left side.

    b. Monitor BP, weight, and urine protein at least every third day.

    c. Assess fetal well-being with fetal movement counts from onset of diagnosis.

    d. Initiate nonstress testing at 37-38 weeks, if indicated.

    e. Consult with physician at first sign of PIH.

    f. Refer for physician management and consideration for hospitalization or delivery at first sign of increasing severity or progression of symptoms.

   g. Follow-up: 6-week postpartum blood pressures should be measured in all women, but particularly in those who had indications of PIH, in order to identify patients with chronic hypertensive disorders.

6. Teaching

   a. Teach woman signs and symptoms indicating progression of the disease and importance of being evaluated immediately if they are present.

   b. Explain physiological benefit of left side-lying and bed rest.

I. Rh-Negative blood type

1. History

   a. Woman's knowledge of her blood type and any previous passive immunization

   b. Exposure history, including transfusion, pregnancy, and childbirth

2. Physical exam: no external characteristics demonstrated

3. Laboratory studies

   a. Blood type

   b. Rh factor

   c. Antibody titer (a sensitized mother will demonstrate a Rh antibody titer greater than 1:8 dilutions)

   d. Antibody identification if titer is positive

4. Differential diagnosis

   a. ABO blood type incompatibilities can cause significant jaundice in newborn.

   b. Kell, Kidd, Duffy, and other antigens are also implicated in newborn jaundice.

5. Management[14]

   a. Repeat antibody screens (with antibody titers and identification if indicated) in third trimester at 26-28 weeks in unsensitized Rh-negative women.

   b. Offer Rh immune globulin (RhoGam) prophylaxis to unsensitized women at 28 weeks gestation.

   c. Order Rh immune globulin (RhoGam) within 72 hours for all unsensitized Rh-negative women who are delivered of an Rh-positive infant, or who have experienced abortion.

   d. Refer to the physician all women with a positive Rh antibody titer for potential management of infant complications.

6. Teaching

   a. Inform woman that Rh status is an inherited factor.

   b. Inform woman of her Rh status, and the events that can lead to subsequent sensitization (Rh antibody formation):

     • Receipt of mismatched blood product

     • Spontaneous and therapeutic abortion

     • Ectopic pregnancy

     • Amniocentesis

       • Partial placenta praevia
       • Marginal abruption
    c. Fully explain benefits and risks of Rh immune globulin prophylaxis.

J. Size-Date discrepancy
1. History
    a. Reconfirm the first day of LNMP.
    b. Reconfirm all other subjective and objective pregnancy dating criteria.
       • Contraceptive use prior to and at time of pregnancy
       • Uterine size at first exam
       • Early pregnancy testing
       • Ultrasonography
       • Quickening and first auscultated fetal heart tones
2. Physical exam
    a. Confirm fundal height measurement by serial assessment; gestational week and centimeter measurement, symphysis to fundus, should be approximately equivalent from 20 to 34 weeks of gestation.
    b. Compare with previously documented pattern of fundal growth.
3. Laboratory studies: ultrasound if discrepancy > 3 cm
4. Differential diagnosis
    a. Size greater than dates
       • Inaccurate gestational age
       • Multiple gestation
       • Macrosomic infant
       • Hydatidiform mole
    b. Size less than dates
       • Inaccurate gestational age
       • Intrauterine growth retardation
       • Fetal abnormalities
       • Oligohydramnios (through spontaneous rupture of membranes or associated with fetal anomaly)
       • Fetal demise
5. Management
    a. Establish new EDC if appropriate.
    b. Consult or refer for identified problems.

K. Toxoplasmosis
1. History
    a. Owner or caretaker of an outdoor cat[51]
    b. Fatigue/malaise
    c. Low grade fever
    d. Sore throat
2. Physical exam: swollen glands in neck
3. Laboratory studies: serum for *Toxoplasma gondii* antibody (two samples, 3 weeks apart)
4. Management[41]

The parasite, once acquired, remains in the body, but becomes dormant. When reactivated or acquired under conditions of a suppressed immune system it can be fatal.

      a. Refer to physician any woman who acquires toxoplasmosis in pregnancy for treatment and abortion counseling as appropriate to the stage of pregnancy and patient's preferences.
      b. Sulfa and antimalarial drugs, in combination, are used to kill the active parasite but have no effect on the dormant stage.
      c. The antimalarial drug pyrimethonine is contraindicated in the first trimester of pregnancy.
      d. Infants of infected mothers should receive treatment in order to reduce the chance of serious complications in later life.
   5. Teaching
      a. Inform at-risk women that transmission is by ingestion of raw or poorly cooked meat from infected animals or by contact with the feces of an infected cat. When the parasite is acquired for the first time during pregnancy, it can be transmitted to the fetus.
      b. Explain that incidence of congenital infection varies with the stage of pregnancy in which the disease is acquired; fewer women pass the infection early in pregnancy but effects to the infant are more damaging at that time.
      c. Instruct woman to avoid handling cat litter. (The cat is the only animal known to excrete *Toxoplasma* in its feces).
      d. Discuss with woman that working in gardens and playing in children's sandboxes are other sources of potential contamination.

L. **Tuberculin test, positive**
   1. History
      a. Previous exposure to tuberculosis organism (family, friends, or work exposure)
      b. Previous disease state
      c. Previous treatment or prophylaxis for the disease
      d. Previous vaccination with *Bacillus* Calmette-Guerin
   2. Physical
      a. A positive reaction is the presence of induration equal to or greater than 10 mm diameter, with or without erythema and tenderness, present 48-72 hours after testing.
      b. A tuberculin skin test becomes positive (10 mm or more) 3-6 weeks after exposure to the tuberculosis organism, which is usually transmitted by the respiratory mode.
   3. Laboratory studies
      a. PPD (purified protein derivative), 0.1 ml antigen injected intradermally
      b. Tine test (old tuberculin[OT]) intracutaneous insertion of antigen carried on multiple metal tines or

    c. Mantoux (PPD or OT): 0.1 ml antigen injected intradermally
4. Differential diagnosis
    a. False-negative reaction occurs during the course of several illnesses, e.g., Hodgkin's disease and measles, therefore, testing should be delayed if these are present.
    b. Persons vaccinated with BCG (*Bacillus* Calmette-Guerin) become tuberculin positive (see below).
5. Management[6, 11]
    a. Conduct a careful patient history to determine recent exposure and family risk.
    b. Do not retest persons who have experienced a previous positive skin test as they may experience severe reactions, with possible necrosis.
    c. Perform chest x-ray with abdominal screening after 20 weeks of pregnancy to rule out active or progressive disease.
    d. Encourage new converters without active disease to receive prophylactic treatment for 1 year with an antituberculin drug such as isoniazid after the first trimester or following delivery.
    e. Refer to physician management patients with radiological evidence of active or inactive disease.
    f. Inform pediatricians of all infants born to mothers with active disease.
    g. Refer all family members and close social contacts of individuals who demonstrate a positive tuberculin response for testing.
    h. Mothers with inactive disease and mothers on prophylactic therapy may breast-feed.
6. Teaching
    a. Discuss importance of screening and treating family members in order to halt transmission of the disease.
    b. Instruct woman to alert all subsequent providers of health care of the positive tuberculin response, and not to accept retesting, in order to prevent an adverse allergen response. Perform chest x-ray if screening is required.

M. Urinary tract infection (UTI)
1. History
    a. Dysuria, frequency, and urgency
    b. Urinary incontinence
    c. Low back pain or pelvic pressure
    d. Suprapubic tenderness
    e. Mild uterine contractions
2. Physical exam
    a. Elicit costovertebral angle (CVA) tenderness.
    b. Palpate abdomen for tenderness and rule out labor.
    c. Take temperature.
3. Laboratory studies
    a. Obtain urinalysis for pyuria (five or more WBCs per field).
    b. Obtain clean catch (mid-stream) urine specimen for culture and iden-

tification of organism (greater than 100,000 bacteria per milliliter of urine) and sensitivity.

4. Differential diagnosis
   a. Preterm labor
   b. Rupture of amniotic membranes
   c. Common discomforts of uterine pressure
5. Management
   a. Consult physician or prescribe antibiotic specific to organism as identified in culture and sensitivity testing.
   b. Immediately prescribe sulfonamides, ampicillin, and/or nitrofurantoins pending results of culture and sensitivity (depending on trimester of pregnancy and patient's allergy to specific drugs), based on history, physical exam, and urinalysis, if available.
   c. Refer febrile woman immediately to physician management.
   d. Consult with physician for all women with history of UTI or pyelonephritis in previous pregnancy for possible antibiotic supression through subsequent pregnancy periods.
   e. Obtain urine cultures in each trimester for women who present with history of asymptomatic bacteruria, urinary infections in previous pregnancies, are positive for sickle-cell trait, or have gestational diabetes.
   f. Repeat urine culture and sensitivity as a test-of-cure following each course of antibiotic therapy for identified infections.
   g. Refer women who develop pyelonephritis in pregnancy for kidney studies after 6 weeks postpartum.
   h. Suggest use of cranberry juice or vitamin C as an ancillary antibacterial agent, as it creates an acidic pH environment in the bladder.
6. Teaching
   a. Encourage frequent emptying of bladder to avoid urine stasis, which promotes bacterial growth.
   b. Increase fluid intake to promote renal function and bladder emptying.
   c. Stress the importance of completing the full course of antibiotic therapy.
   d. Advise that personal hygiene (wiping front to back) helps reduce colonization of fecal *Bacillus* from rectum to urethra.
   e. Advise that voiding after intercourse helps to reduce UTIs cross-colonized from oral and genital tracts.

N. **Vaginal bleeding**
1. History
   a. Amount and characteristics of bleeding
   b. Relationship of bleeding events to activity (work, intercourse, exercise)
   c. Gestational age
   d. Obstetrical history, including previous bleeding events
   e. Concurrent abdominal pain or cramping or pelvic pressure
2. Physical exam
   a. Obtain vital signs (BP and pulse).

b. Perform abdominal exam.
c. Auscultate fetal heart tones as appropriate.
d. Clinical features will vary, depending on etiology of the vaginal bleeding.
   - Abortion
     — Wide variation in amount of bleeding
     — Uterine tenderness may be present
     — Cramping, with or without passage of tissue
   - Abruptio placenta
     — Rigid boardlike abdomen
     — Irritable/tender uterus
     — Absence of fetal heart tones (possible)
     — Signs and symptoms of impending maternal shock
   - Bloody "show"
     — Signs and symptoms of early latent phase of labor
   - Cervicitis or cervical polyps
     — Signs and symptoms of concomitant vaginitis
     — Observation of pedunculated and vascular tissue masses adherent to cervix
   - Ectopic pregnancy (ruptured)
     — Severe abdominal pain: may radiate to shoulder, may be unilateral
     — Progressive symptoms of blood loss, can progress to the shock state
   - Hydatidiform mole
     — Severe nausea and vomiting
     — Uterus larger than dates, without documentation of fetal skeleton or fetal heart tones
     — Early development of signs of toxemia of pregnancy
   - Placenta praevia
     — Silent vaginal bleeding
     — Unengaged presenting part, near or at term
     — Abnormal fetal position (possible)
3. Laboratory assessment: order tests as indicated by stage of pregnancy and suspected causes of vaginal bleeding to diagnose and/or to rule out the following:
   a. Pregnancy
   b. Degree of maternal physiological adaptation to blood loss
4. Differential diagnosis
   a. Uterine
      - Abortion—threatened, inevitable, incomplete, or complete
      - Abruptio placenta
      - Bloody show
      - Ectopic pregnancy
      - Hydatidiform mole
      - placenta praevia

   b. Cervical
      • Cervicitis
      • Cervical trauma or cervical polyps
   c. Vaginal trauma
   d. Malignancy (cervical or uterine)
   e. Abdominal emergencies (appendicitis, bowel torsion, rupture, or torsion of ovarian cysts) will not present with vaginal bleeding but must be considered as a source of pain
5. Management
   a. Before 20 weeks gestation
      • Obtain detailed menstrual and obstetrical history.
      • Obtain urine HCG if any doubt of pregnancy.
      • Obtain serum HCG if suspicious of abortion or ectopic pregnancy.
      • Perform gentle speculum examination to identify source of bleeding.
      • Treat identified vaginitis or cervicitis as indicated by trimester of pregnancy.
      • Order "pelvic rest" for all causes of threatened abortion or vascular cervical polyps, i.e., avoid digital and speculum examination, vaginal medicinal therapies, and sexual intercourse.
      • Refer women who experience incomplete or "missed" (retained products of gestation) abortions for evacuation of uterine content.
      • Refer women experiencing acute abdominal discomfort for the immediate assessment of acute abdominal emergencies, e.g., ruptured ectopic pregnancy.
      • Refer to physician management women suspected of molar pregnancy.
   b. After 20 weeks gestation
      • Order sonographic evaluation for placental localization.
      • Prescribe pelvic rest: avoid digital and speculum examination, vaginal medicinal therapies, and sexual intercourse.
      • Refer all women experiencing silent vaginal bleeding and/or acute abdominal pain for immediate diagnosis and management by physician.
6. Teaching
   a. Provide teaching as appropriate to the suspected cause of bleeding and stage of pregnancy.
   b. Grief counseling may be indicated and appropriate as anticipatory guidance in cases of abortion and/or fetal death.
O. **Vaginitis**: the various organisms that cause vaginitis in the well-woman gynecological phases of the life cycle can also affect the pregnant patient; diagnosis and treatment of these conditions in the pregnant patient can be found in Chapter 2.

VI. Antepartal assessment of fetal well-being

A. Fetal movement count: fetal movements are any type or variety of fetal activity in vivo perceived by the mother; more than 10 fetal movements in a 12-hour period are associated with fetal well-being. Decreased fetal activity or cessation of fetal activity can be predictive of fetal distress, and should be investigated.

   1. Indications[16]

     a. Fetal movement records can be kept by all women, at any stage of pregnancy (Appendix A).

     b. Fetal movement records should be kept by women in all high-risk pregnancy categories.

   2. Teaching

     a. Report a marked decrease in fetal activity to the health care provider.

     b. Immediately report any count of fetal movement less than 10 in a 12-hour period.

B. Non-Stress Testing (NST): nonstress testing is the assessment of fetal heart rate, fetal movement, and fetal heart rate acceleration using electronic (usual) or auscultated (in research) external monitoring devices. A reactive NST (the desired result) is one in which there are two or more adequate FHR accelerations (15 beats per minute above baseline, lasting 15 seconds or more) during a 10-20 minute test period.[14,19,39,44] (Note: Current sources vary widely on this definition, ranging from two to four fetal movements, 10-40-minute observation period, 10-15 bpm acceleration.)

   1. Indications for testing

     a. All reports of decreased fetal movement

     b. All women at 42 weeks of gestational age

     c. Women in selected high risk pregnancy categories should be tested weekly from 36 weeks gestation

       • Maternal diabetes

       • Intrauterine growth retardation

       • Hypertension

   2. Teaching

     a. Instruct woman that the nonstress test is a screening procedure used as an adjunct to other measures of the determination of fetal well-being.

     b. Instruct woman that a "reactive test" is associated with fetal well-being, but that it must be repeated at least weekly for continued validity.

C. Contraction stress testing (CST): the CST is an assessment of fetal heart rate under conditions of naturally occurring, naturally induced (nipple stimulation) or artifically induced (oxytocin) uterine contractions using an external monitoring device. A negative CST (the desired result) is one in which at least three uterine contractions are measured in a 10-minute period, during which the fetus manifests a normal baseline heart rate without evidence of late deceleration. A suspicious result is one in which there are any decelerations that are not persistent. A positive result is one in which late decelerations are coincident with more than 50 percent of contractions.

   1. Indications for the test

     a. All women who have demonstrated a nonreactive nonstress test

b. Women with demonstrated IUGR (perform from time of diagnosis weekly to time of delivery)

c. Women in selected high risk categories, on an individualized basis.

Women who prefer to exhaust "natural" therapies before medicinal intervention may prefer the breast-stimulation CST.

---

2. Teaching
   a. Exogenous CST
      • Inform woman that a negative CST is associated with fetal well-being, but must be repeated at least weekly for continued validity.
      • Woman should maintain daily fetal movement count charts as a helpful adjunct to confirming fetal well-being.
   b. Endogenous CST (breast-stimulation CST)
      • Implications of a negative endogenous CST are equivalent to those of the exogenous test.
      • Teach woman and/or partner to roll one nipple from 1-2 minutes, followed by a 5-minute rest period. Repeat on the alternate side (instructions vary).[14]
      • Teach woman to stop nipple stimulation at the onset of a uterine contraction.
      • BSCST is not recommended in out-of-hospital settings because of a potential for hypertonic uterine response. Prolonged, tetanic contractions, or contractions occurring more frequently than every 3 minutes, indicate need to interrupt the stimulation sequence.
      • Inform woman that a negative BSCST is associated with fetal well-being, but must be repeated at least weekly for continued validity.
D. Ultrasonography: ultrasonography is the visualization of the intrauterine environment using sonic devices and may include the concurrent qualitative or quantitative measurement of fetal well-being (the biophysical profile).
   1. Indications (according to NIH Consensus Development Conference Report[17])
      a. To determine gestational age for women with uncertain dates or for those scheduled to undergo elective termination of pregnancy
      b. As an adjunct to special procedures, e.g., amniocentesis
      c. To evaluate the fetal condition in all cases of clinical size-date discrepancies, including diagnosis and management of multiple gestations, growth retardation, and poly-or oligohydramnios
      d. To evaluate the fetal condition in mothers of selected high risk pregnancy categories: use serially throughout the course of pregnancy
      e. For placental localization in case of vaginal bleeding
      f. To determine fetal presentation, as an adjunct to clinical management, e.g., breech version
      g. To obtain a biophysical profile of all fetuses at 42 weeks of gestation.
   2. Management and teaching[12,29]

      a. Inform woman that current data suggest no adverse effects of ultra-sonography on the developing fetus, at human dosage levels, but long term effects have not yet been determined.

      b. Instruct woman to drink three to four 8-ounce glasses of water 1 hour prior to the procedure in order to have a full bladder (if ultrasound is done early in gestation or for placental localization).

      c. Discuss results with woman.

      d. For women having ultrasound for amniocentesis, be sensitive to bonding that can take place while parents visualize the fetus on monitor since some may need to elect to terminate the pregnancy.

E. Amniocentesis: amniocentesis is the aspiration of amniotic fluid from the uterine cavity.

  1. Indications

      a. In second trimester

        • For identification of genetic (chromosomal) structures

        • For analysis of selected amniotic fluid substrates, e.g., alpha-fetoprotein and metabolic enzymes.

      b. In developing gestations, perform for diagnosis and therapy of affected infants, e.g., Rh-affected fetuses

      c. In late gestation, for determination of fetal lung maturity.

  2. Management and teaching

      a. Inform women who have indications for amniocentesis that approximately 200 tests can be performed on amniotic fluid samples for diagnosis of various fetal conditions.

      b. Inform woman that the risks associated with amniocentesis are less than 1 percent.

        • Possible spontaneous abortion

        • Uterine infection

        • Bleeding

      c. Document counseling, including pregnancy options, at various gestational ages.

      d. Document counseling given to all mothers 35 years of age and older.

      e. Discuss with Rh-negative unsensitized mothers that they may wish to accept administration of Rh immune globulin to avert sensitization as a consequence of the procedure.

VII. Guidelines for common concerns in pregnancy

A. Alcohol[24,50,57]

  1. Alcohol ingested by the mother is transported across the placenta.

  2. Ingestion of 1-3 or more ounces of absolute alcohol each day places the fetus at definite risk of being born with "fetal alcohol syndrome" which is characterized by prenatal or postnatal growth retardation, congenital abnormalities, central nervous system abnormality, and newborn alcoholic dependency, with developmental delay.

3. Best advice is *don't drink*.
4. Additional adverse pregnancy outcomes associated with alcohol are as follows:
   a. Spontaneous abortion
   b. Lowered birth weight
   c. Preterm delivery
   d. Intrauterine growth retardation
   e. Abnormal neurobehavioral and neural development

B. Employment[43]
   1. There are few restrictions on employment within the framework of several reasonable precautions:
      a. Prolonged standing should be avoided, and several rest periods for elevation of the legs and feet should be integrated into the work schedule.
      b. Heavy lifting is contraindicated.
   2. Occupations that require balance may be contraindicated in later pregnancy.
   3. Exposure to occupational health risks such as toxic substances (e.g., benzene, chlorinated hydrocarbons, lead compounds, mercury, and several inhaled anesthetic agents), excessive noise, and radiation should be avoided throughout pregnancy and may be of particular concern in early gestation.

C. Exercise[3,18,36]
   1. Exercise in moderation is to be encouraged. Maternal heart rate should not exceed 70 percent maximum efficiency (220 minus the maternal age times 0.7), or 140 beats/minute maximum.
   2. Strenuous exercise should not exceed 15 minutes in duration.
   3. Exercise should not be performed from the supine position after the 4th month of pregnancy.
   4. Adequate hydration during and after exercise is essential.
   5. Women should be aware of excessive uterine activity (four to five contractions in an hour) following exercise.
   6. Stretching and toning are as important in pregnancy as at any other period. Warm up and cool down periods are essential.
   7. Strenuous sports that involve jarring motions and sports that require balance may present difficulties later in pregnancy.
   8. Scuba diving below one atmosphere and parachuting should be avoided due to changes in atmospheric pressure.

D. Medication and drug use
   1. Several over-the-counter (OTC) medications (at excessive doses), prescription drugs, and illegal drug substances are known teratogenic agents. Health care providers should inquire of woman's OTC medication practices.
   2. All drug ingestion should be avoided in the first trimester. (Risks and benefits of essential therapeutic medications must be acknowledged.)
   3. Data continue to be evaluated regarding effects of marijuana and several

other illegal substances. Heroin and cocaine are associated with increased risk of abortion, congenital malformation, and prematurity. Narcotic addiction of the newborn is possible.[4,7]

4. Aspirin should be avoided due to prolongation of bleeding time in the mother. Close to term aspirin should be avoided also because of its potential fetal effects of increased bleeding time and jaundice (due to competition with bilirubin for albumin binding). An acetaminophen product is preferable if analgesic effect is required.

E. Sexual relations
   1. Sexual arousal will vary as a consequence of the developmental stage of pregnancy and may differ among women.[38]
   2. In general, coitus and orgasm are not contraindicated, as long as amniotic membranes are intact, and there is no placenta praevia or symptoms of preterm labor.[32]
   3. Specific prohibitions against coitus and orgasm may be indicated in the following:
      a. Pelvic or abdominal pain
      b. Preterm labor, or history of preterm labor
      c. Ruptured membranes
      d. Threatened abortion
      e. Undiagnosed vaginal bleeding
   4. Alternative sexual positions may be desirable in later pregnancy to avoid abdominal pressure.

F. Smoking
   1. Smoking has adverse effects on both intra- and extrauterine environments.[45]
   2. Infants born of women who smoke weigh less than infants of mothers who do not smoke.
   3. Smoking increases the risk of spontaneous abortion and preterm labor.
   4. Pregnant smokers should be encouraged to stop or at least decrease the quantity of cigarettes smoked each day.

G. Spas, saunas, and general bathing
   1. Immersion in very hot tub water or sauna should not exceed a period of 15 minutes. Maternal core temperature should not exceed 102° F. Intrauterine fetal body temperature is also raised by such immersion.
   2. Regular bathing is not contraindicated, although the imbalance of late pregnancy requires caution and prudent assistance in entering and exiting the tub or shower.

H. Travel
   1. Travel is not generally restricted at any stage in pregnancy; however, it may not be advisable after the 36th week if considerable distance is contemplated.
   2. Shorter periods of travel with frequent rest and stretch stops are advisable to forestall edema and fatigue.
   3. Snacks and fluids should be available when needed by the traveler.

4. Extra fluid intake and avoidance of caffeine beverages, will limit dehydration during air travel.
5. A copy of the prenatal chart should accompany the traveler in the event of the need for emergency care.
6. Air travel may be interdicted by the airline in the last month of pregnancy, by company policy.

I. Vaccinations
1. Live or attenuated virus vaccines can be teratogenic in early pregnancy.[38]
2. Killed virus vaccines can be given, if indicated.
3. Children of a pregnant mother may be vaccinated.

Teratogen information programs are a good source of information and can be called by patient or provider for current information and counseling recommendations (see Appendix B).

VIII. Guidelines for antepartum care in alternative settings

The following information is offered as a guideline for health care practitioners who provide birthing services in out-of-hospital settings. The factors identified are suggested as a basis for low- versus high- risk assignment. Site-specific criteria should be developed and adapted appropriately for the population served in any geographic setting.

A. Preexisting factors that would exclude a woman from being considered for out-of-hospital delivery:
1. Sociodemographic characteristics[26]
   a. Age
      • less than 17
      • more than 40 and nulliparous
      • more than 45 and multiparous
   b. Residence: distance of residence from site of antepartum care
   c. Substance abuse: current ingestion and/or unwillingness to terminate use of mind-altering drugs, tobacco, or alcohol
2. Maternal medical history
   a. Cardiovascular system
      • Congenital heart defects
      • Cardiac disease
      • Chronic hypertension
      • Pulmonary embolus
   b. Endocrine system
      • Diabetes mellitus
      • Thyroid disease
      • Lupus erythymatosis or autoimmune disease
   c. Hematopoietic system

- Anemia of congenital origin (e.g., thalassemia, sickle cell disease)
- Bleeding disorders
  d. Neurological system
- Documented psychotic disorder previously treated
- Current mental health problem with medication management
- Epilepsy, with or without current use of anticonvulsive medication
- Paralysis, muscular or neurological origin
  e. Respiratory system
- Asthma
- Chronic bronchitis
- Tuberculosis
  f. Skeletal system: skeletal deformity of lumbar or pelvic regions
  g. Urologic system
- Pyelonephritis
- Renal disease (nephritis or chronic renal insufficiency)
3. Maternal obstetrical history
  a. Abortion
- Three or more spontaneous or therapeutic abortions
- One septic abortion
  b. Abruptio placenta
  c. Antibody screen positive
- Previous Rh sensitization
- Presence of Kell, Kidd or Duffy or other antibodies causing hemolytic disease
  d. Birthweight < 2500 g or > 4000 g
  e. Genetic or metabolic disorder of previous infant
  f. Gestational diabetes
  g. Hypertensive disorder
  h. Major congenital malformations of previous infant
  i. Parity of five or more
  j. Placenta praevia or third trimester bleeding
  k. Postpartum hemorrhage
  l. Stillbirth (> 28 weeks gestation)
  m. Uterine surgery, including previous cesarean section
4. Maternal physical status and laboratory findings
  a. Advanced gestational age: seeking antepartum care late in pregnancy
  b. Obesity
  c. Cardiac murmur
- Systolic murmur equal to or greater than grade 3
- Diastolic murmur
  d. Anemia (Hct equal to or less than 32 percent)
B. Factors that may develop during pregnacy that would exclude a woman from being considered for out-of-hospital delivery.
  1. Socioeconomic characteristics
  a. Noncompliance with mutually determined plan of care

     b. Substance abuse

     c. Unsuitability of the home for delivery, as determined following site visit

  2. Maternal physical status

     a. Cardiovascular system

- Development of symptoms of cardiac insufficiency
- Progressive development of varicosities in pelvis or extremities
- Thrombophlebitis
- Development of PIH

     b. Endocrine system

- Development of gestational diabetes
- Progression of thyroid enlargment beyond normal pregnancy limits

     c. Respiratory system: acute asthma

     d. Neurologic system

- Symptoms of emerging psychotic instability
- Onset of paralysis e.g., Guillain-Barré syndrome

     e. Hematopoietic system: anemia unresponsive to oral iron supplementation (Hct less than or equal to 30 percent at 37 weeks of gestation).

     f. Urologic system—pyelonephritis

     g. Other findings

- Abnormal weight gain
  - < 12 pounds total
  - > 50 pounds total
- Abnormal laboratory findings
  - Onset of Rh sensitization or rise in any identified antibody titer
  - Acute viral or bacterial disease that compromises neonatal status
  - Evidence of herpetic lesion or positive culture at 36 weeks gestation or thereafter

  3. Maternal obstetrical status

     a. Abortion: complete, incomplete, or missed

     b. Amniocentesis, positive for fetal chromosomal or genetic disorder

     c. Abruptio placenta or praevia

     d. Estimated fetal weight > 9 pounds

     e. Intrauterine growth retardation

     f. Multiple gestation

     g. Nonvertex presentation at or beyond 37 weeks of gestation

     h. Postdates (42 weeks)

     i. Vaginal bleeding

REFERENCES

1. Abrams M: Health care for women. J Obstet Gynecol Neonatal Nurs 15(3):250-255, 1986

2. Adams C (ed): Nurse-Midwifery: Health Care for Women and Newborns. Orlando, FL, Grune & Stratton, 1983
3. Artal R, Wiswell R, Romen Y, et al: Pulmonary responses to exercise in pregnancy. Am J Obstet Gynecol 154:378-383,1986
4. Asch RH, Smith CE: Effects of marijuana on reproduction. Contemp Obstet Gynecol 19:217, 1982
5. Bates B: A Guide to Physical Examination (ed 4). Philadelphia, Lippincott, 1987
6. Beare P, Rahr V, Ronshausen C: Nursing Implications of Diagnostic Tests. Philadelphia, Lippincott, 1985
7. Berkowitz R, Coustan D, Mochizuki T: Handbook for Prescribing Medications During Pregnancy. Boston, Little, Brown, 1981
8. Bishop E, Cefalo R: Signs and Symptoms in Disorders in Pregnancy. Philadelphia, Lippincott, 1983
9. Boehme T: Hepatitis B: The nurse-midwife's role in management and prevention. J Nurse-Midwifery 30(2):79-87, 1985
10. Brucker M, Macmillen N: What's new in pregnancy tests. J Obstet Gynecol Neonatal Nurs 14(5):353-359, 1985
11. Bush J: Protocol for tuberculosis screening in pregnancy. J Obstet Gynecol Neonatal Nurs 15(3):225-230, 1986
12. Campbell S, et al: Ultrasound scanning in pregnancy: short-term psychologic effects of early real-time scans. J Psychosom Obstet Gynecol I-2:57-61, 1982
13. CDC: Hepatitis. Hepatitis Surveillance Report, Washington, DC, U.S. Department of Health and Human Services, 47-8-40, 1981.
14. Creasy R, Resnik R: Maternal Fetal Medicine. Philadelphia, Saunders, 1984
15. D'Alamo R, Lee R, Pa-In K, et al: Intestinal parasites in pregnancy. Obstet Gynecol 66:639, 1985
16. Davis L: Daily fetal movement counting: A valuable assessment tool. J Nurse-Midwifery, 32(1):11-19, 1987
17. Diagnostic Ultrasound Imaging in Pregnancy. National Institutes of Health Consensus Development Conference. Consensus Statement, Vol. 5, No. 1. Washington, DC, U.S. Department of Health and Human Services, 1984
18. Fogel I, Woods N: Health Care of Women: A Nursing Perspective. St. Louis, Mosby, 1981
19. Freeman R, Garrite T: Fetal Heart Rate Monitoring. Baltimore, Williams & Wilkins, 1981
20. Gabbe S: Definition, detection, and management of gestational diabetes. Obstet Gynecol 67(1):121-124, 1986
21. Hobel C: Risk assessment in perinatal medicine. Clin Obstet Gynecol 21(2):287-295, 1978
22. Jones J, Cox A, Levy E: Women's Health Management: Guidelines for Nurse-practitioners. Reston, VA, Publishing, 1984
23. Levin M, Rigg L, Marshall R: Pregnancy and diabetes. Arch Intern Med 146:758-767, 1986

24. Little R, Asker R, Sampson P, et al: Fetal growth and moderate drinking in early pregnancy. Am J Epidemiol 123(2): 270-278, 1986
25. Loreman A: AIDS in pregnancy. J Obstet Gynecol Neonatal Nurs 15(2):91-93, 1986
26. Lubic R: Evaluation of an out-of-hospital maternity center for low-risk patients, in Aiken L (ed) Health Policy and Nursing Practice. New York, McGraw-Hill, 1980
27. Malasanos L, Barkauskas V, Moss M, et al:Health Assessment. St Louis: Mosby, 1986
28. Maternal and Child Health Branch, California Department of Health Services: Nutrition During Pregnancy and the Postpartum Period. (Review Draft 8/1/87) Sacramento, CA: California Department of Health Services (in press)
29. Mole R: Possible hazards of imaging and doppler ultrasound in obstetrics. Birth 13(1):29-38, 1986
30. Neeson J, May K: Comprehensive Maternity Nursing. Philadelphia, Lippincott, 1986
31. Neeson J, Stockdale C: The Practitioner's Handbook of Ambulatory Ob/Gyn. New York, Wiley and Sons, 1981
32. Neilson J: Indications for ultrasonography in obstetrics. Birth 13(1):16-20, 1986
33. Neural Tube Defects, (informational pamphlet). American College of Obstetricians and Gynecologists, 1985, Washington, DC
34. Oskowitz S: Elderly gravida. in Friedman E (ed): Obstetrical Decision Making. St. Louis, Mosby, 1982, pp 14-15
35. Perkins RP. (1979). Sexual behavior and response in relation to complications of pregnancy. Am J Obstet Gynecol 134:498, 1979
36. Pregnancy and Postnatal Exercise Guidelines (informational pamphlet). Washington, DC, American College of Obstetrics and Gynecology.
37. Principles of nutrition and dietary recommendations for individuals with diabetes mellitus. *Diabetes*, 28:1027, 1979
38. Postotnik P: Drugs and pregnancy in FDA Consumer. Department of Health and Human Services Publication # (FDA) 80-3083, Washington, DC, U.S. Government Printing Office,1978.
39. Rayburn W, Lavin J: Obstetrics for the House Officer. Baltimore, Williams & Wilkins, 1984
40. Roberts J: Priorities in prenatal education. J Obstet Gynecol Neonatal Nurs, 5(3):17-20, 1976
41. Romney S, Gray M, Little A, et al: Gynecology and Obstetrics: The Health Care of Women. New York, McGraw Hill, 1981
42. Root B, King J: Environmental influences in fetal development, maternal nutrition, in Creasy R, Resnik R (eds): Maternal Fetal Medicine. Philadelphia, WB Saunders, 1984
43. Saurel-Cubizolles M J, Kiniski M: Work in pregnancy: Its evolving relationship with perinatal outcome. A review. Social Sci Med 22(4):431-442, 1986

44. Schrifrin B, Foye G, Amato J: Routine fetal heart rate monitoring in the antepartum period. Obstet Gynecol 54:21-25, 1979
45. Shiono P, Klebanoff M, Rhoads G: Smoking and drinking during pregnancy. JAMA 255(1): 82-83, 1986
46. Sonstegard L, Kowalski K, Jennings B: Women's Health, Volume I: Ambulatory Care. Orlando, FL, Grune & Stratton, 1982
47. Sonstegard L, Kowalski K, Jennings B: Women's Health, Volume II: Childbearing. Orlando, FL, Grune & Stratton, 1983
48. Stagno S, Whitley R: Current concepts: Herpesvirus infections of pregnancy: Part II-Herpes simplex virus and varicella-zoster virus infections. N Engl J Med 313:1270,1274,1327-1330, 1985
49. Summary and recommendations of the second international workshop-Conference on gestational diabetes mellitus. (1985). Diabetes, 34:(Suppl 2)
50. The effects of alcohol on pregnancy outcome. Alcohol Health and Research World 9(1):Fall, 1984.
51. Toxoplasmosis, NIH Publication #83-308, Sept. 1983, U.S. Department of Health and Human Services.
52. Whitley, N. (1985). A Manual of Clinical Obstetrics. Philadelphia: J.B. Lippincott Company.
53. Willis, J. Genetic Counseling: Learning What to Expect. Department of Health and Human Services, Publication #(FDA) 81-9006. U.S. Government Printing Office, September 1980.
54. Willis, J. All about eating for two. Department of Health and Human Services, Publication #(FDA) 84-2183. U.S. Government Printing Office, March 1984.
55. Willard, M: The educational pelvic examination: women's responses to a new approach. J Obstet Gynecol Neonatal Nurs (March/April), 135-139, 1986
56. Worthington-Roberts B, Vermeersch J. Williams S: Nutrition in Pregnancy and Lactation. St. Louis, Time/Mirror/Mosby, 1985
57. Wright, J. (1986). Alcohol in pregnancy. Brit J Obstet Gynecol 93:201-202, 1985

APPENDIX A: FETAL MOVEMENT RECORD

We would like you to keep a record of how often your baby moves. All babies should move every day. Some babies move a lot, while other babies move a little. Each baby is different. You should count the number of times your baby moves and record it on the chart. You should do this every day until you are told to stop or until your baby is born. Keep this record with you. Bring it to each prenatal visit and whenever you go to the hospital for any reason.

Directions

At 9:00 A.M., start counting the number of times your baby moves. each day. Each time your baby moves, put a mark next to the closest time. When your baby has moved 10 times, stop counting for that day. Color in the time box when you stopped counting. If for some reason you can not start counting at 9:00 A.M., write the time you did start counting in the "time started" box for that particular day.

Important: Go immediately to the hospital if you do not feel any movement in 8 hours, or if you have not felt ten (10) movements in 12 hours. Be sure to take a copy of the record with you to the hospital.

FETAL MOVEMENT RECORD

Name: _____   Clinic: _____   Birthdate: _____   EDC: _____

Date: _____   Weeks: _____   Weeks: _____

*Time Started	Mon	Tues	Weds	Thurs	Fri	Sat	Sun	Mon	Tues	Weds	Thurs	Fri	Sat	Sun
9:00														
9:30														
10:00														
10:30														
11:00														
11:30														
12:00														
12:30														
1:00														
1:30														
2:00														
2:30														
3:00														
3:30														
4:00														
4:30														

138

	Mon	Tues	Weds	Thurs	Fri	Sat	Sun	Mon	Tues	Weds	Thurs	Fri	Sat	Sun
5:00														
5:30														
6:00														
6:30														
7:00														
7:30														
8:00														
8:30														
9:00														
Total														

*Please write the time you started counting in the box (if it was not at 9:00 a.m.)

APPENDIX B: TERATOGEN INFORMATION PROGRAMS

Arizona Teratogen Information
  Network
Tucson, Arizona
602-626-6016
800-362-0101 (in Arizona)

Califormia Teratogen Registry
San Deigo, California
619-294-3581
800-532-3749 (in California)

Connecticut Pregnancy Exposure
  Information Service
Farmington, Connecticut
203-674-2676
800-325-5391 (in Connecticut)

Teratology Program
Miami, Florida
305-547-6006

Iowa Teratogen Information Center
Iowa City, Iowa
319-356-2674

Pregnancy/Environmental Hotline
Brighton, Massachusetts
617-787-4957
800-322-5104 (Massachusetts)

FDA Adverse Drug Effects Branch
Rockville, Maryland
301-443-6410

Teratology Service Network
Camden, New Jersey
609-757-7869

Pregnancy Healthline
New York, New York
212-230-1111

Pregnancy Healthline
Philadelphia, Pennsylvania
215-829-KIDS

Pregnancy Safety Hotline
Pitsburgh, Pennsylvania
412-687-SAFE

Genetic Screening and Counseling
  Service
Denton, Texas
817-383-3561

Teratogen Identification Program
Houston, Texas
713-792-4592

Pregnancy Risk Line
Salt Lake City, Utah
801-583-2229 (in Utah and
  Montana only)

Vermont Teratogen Information
  Network
Burlington, Vermont
802-658-4310

Drug Information Service
Seattle, Washington
206-543-3373

Wisconsin Teratogen Project
Madison, Wisconsin
608-262-9722
800-362-3020 (in Wisconsin)

Teratology Hotline
Milwaukee, Wisconsin
414-931-4172

Reproduction Toxicology Center
Washington, DC
202-293-5137 (for members only; call
  for information of joining)

Motherisk
Toronto, Ontario
Canada
416k-598-5781

Chapter 6

Intrapartum Assessment and Management

Vanda R. Lops   *Mary K. Barger*

I. Initial assessment

A. History (from review of prenatal record or from mother).
   1. Obtain sociodemographic information:
     a. Name
     b. Age (teens and elderly gravidas may be at greater risk for certain conditions)
     c. Marital status
     d. Childbirth education
     e. Support during labor
     f. Sociocultural background
     g. Specific stress factors in self or environment as noted in chart
     h. Mother's desires for her labor and delivery experience
   2. Ascertain gravidity and parity.
   3. Assess gestational age.
     a. Last menstrual period (LNMP)
     b. Early exam confirming congruency of size and LMP
     c. When fetal heart tones first auscultated by fetoscope and number of weeks documented fetal heart tones
     d. Sonogram (done for gestational age)
   4. Review antepartum course.
     a. Abnormalities noted on initial physical
     b. Abnormal lab studies
       • Positive antibody screen
       • Presence of anemia
       • Presence of infectious diseases, including syphilis, gonorrhea, hepatitis, herpes, human immundeficiency virus (HIV), and *Chlamydia*, and appropriate follow up
       • Positive urine cultures and follow-up
     c. Total weight gain and nutritional status
     d. Fundal growth and any studies, if results not normal

    e. Blood pressure, urine, and edema at each visit

    f. Any problems or complications noted and their treatment or ongoing management

5. Review family history and mother's medical-surgical history for factors that may affect intrapartum or postpartum care.

6. Review past obstetric history:
   a. Pregnancy complications
   b. Length of labor
   c. Gestational age at delivery
   d. Type of delivery
   e. Weight of largest baby versus smallest
   f. Any postpartum complications

7. Elicit mother's chief complaint including description, onset, signs, and symptoms and any associated factors.

8. If labor is suspected, question mother further:
   a. Status of uterine contractions
      - Time of onset of regular uterine contractions
      - Location and radiation
      - Intensity
      - Frequency
      - Duration
      - Influence of position change on character of contractions
   b. Status of membranes, if ruptured: time of rupture and color and amount of fluid.
   c. Presence of show for amount, consistency, and color (rule out frank bleeding)
   d. Presence and amount of fetal movement

B. Physical exam

1. Observe mother for the following:
   a. Facial expression and position of body
   b. Verbal behavior (what she says about how she is feeling)
   c. Respirations, e.g., rate, holding breath, "catch in breath," grunting
   d. Physical activity, e.g., frequency of movement, lack of movement, bearing down
   e. Ability to respond to supportive or coaching measures

2. Note vital signs.

3. Palpate abdomen for the following:
   a. Uterine contractions: frequency, duration, intensity (electronic monitor tracing can confirm frequency and duration)
   b. Fundal height in centimeters
   c. Contour and condition of abdominal wall, i.e., fibroids, undue uterine tenderness, scars

5. Fetal heart rate per auscultation or external fetal monitor tracing (rate, baseline, accelerations, or decelerations)

6. Fetal activity as felt by examiner.

7. Perform Leopold maneuvers for the following:
   a. Presentation, position, and attitude of baby
   b. Station of presenting part
   c. Estimated fetal weight
8. Perform pelvic evaluation.
   a. Observe perineum for the following:
      - Show
      - Frank bleeding
      - Lesions
      - Gross leaking of amniotic fluid (note color)
      - Signs of perineal/rectal pressure with or without contractions
      - Signs and symptoms of stage II labor:
        — Opening of vaginal canal
        — Bulging of perineum
        — Passage of flatus or fecal matter
        — Flattening of rectum
        — Exposed or everted rectal mucosa
        — Visible caput
   b. Perform pelvic examination for the following:
      - Cervical effacement
      - Cervical dilation
      - Fetal presentation
      - Station and position of presenting part
      - Status of membranes (in absence of history or suspicion of spontaneous rupture)
      - Assess rectum for fullness
   c. Perform speculum exam as necessary for the following:
      - Diagnosis of spontaneous rupture of membranes
      - Culture of cervix if necessary, e.g., in preterm labor
      - Visualization of vagina and cervix for any lesions (as with history of herpes)
      - Identification of source of vaginal bleeding when ultrasound shows no previa or low-lying placenta
9. Evaluate other systems and perform branching examinations as appropriate to chief complaint or other problems elicited from history.
C. Laboratory studies
   1. Perform dipstick urine for protein and glucose.
   2. Test for spontaneous rupture of membranes (see Section V, I).
   3. If patient is admitted, do the following:
      a. Obtain hemoglobin (Hgb) or hematocrit (Hct).
      b. Perform or order urinalysis.
      c. Obtain blood for type and screen (may not be done in all settings).
D. Management and teaching
   1. Discharge undelivered.
      a. Appropriate candidates are the following:

- Those not in labor
- Those in latent phase who prefer to wait for active phase at home
- Those whose chief complaint is resolved, e.g., rupture of membranes is ruled out
- Those whose exam and fetal status are normal

  b. Instruct the woman regarding the following:
  - Signs and symptoms of labor
  - Immediate return if she has vaginal bleeding, rupture of membranes, sudden increase in signs of labor, or any other problems for which she deems evaluation is necessary
  - Availability of provider by telephone if she has any questions
  - Ingestion of complex carbohydrates (no fat; low protein) and clear fruit juices if in early labor
  - Normal course of labor and comfort measures for early labor.

2. Encourage the woman to ambulate prior to formal admission if in hospital setting.
   a. Appropriate candidates are the following:
   - Those in whom the diagnosis of false labor versus early labor is in doubt, especially multiparas
   - Those who live far from the birth setting
   - Those with significant cervical dilation but hypotonic contraction pattern
   - Those with good fetal status (reactive nonstress test, negative endogenous contraction stress test, or reassuring fetal heart rate pattern)

   b. Make sure that the woman is appropriately attired.
   c. Attempt to have someone walk with the woman or, if this is impossible, frequently check on her.
   d. Instruct the woman regarding the following:
   - Appropriate areas in which to ambulate
   - To return immediately if rupture of membranes occurs
   - To return if contractions increase in frequency and duration

   e. Reexamine the woman in 1-2 hours per practitioner judgement

3. Admit or decide to stay with the woman (dependent on birth setting).
   a. Perform and document general physical examination, practitioner assessment, and plan of management. (This is a requirement in hospitals and the standard of practice in out-of-hospital birth sites.)
   b. Order or perform appropriate laboratory tests (see section I, C, 3).
   c. Write admission orders as appropriate.
   d. Inform physician of mother's status as per protocol.
   e. Consult with physician if woman is less than 37 weeks or greater than 42 weeks gestation.

II. Management of stage I

A. Ongoing assessment of maternal status[25]
  1. Maintain adequate hydration and energy level.

a. Offer clear liquids as tolerated: minimum 4 ounces per hour.
b. Initiate intravenous fluids at not more than 100 ml/hr [6,11]or set up venous access in the following cases:
  • If the woman is dehydrated, especially with severe ketonuria present
  • If there is a history of previous labor complications, e.g., postpartum hemorrhage or uterine inversion
  • In high-risk patients, e.g., those with a large baby, multiple gestation, polyhydramnios, anemia, or grand multiparity

2. Monitor blood pressure, pulse, and respirations every hour. Take temperature every 4 hours. Increase frequency of vital sign assessment as dictated by mother's condition.
3. Assess bladder periodically and encourage frequent voiding; if the mother has not voided in 6-8 hours or if a distended bladder palpated, catheterize with straight catheter.
4. Maintain the mother's hygiene, including the following:
  a. Showering or bathing during long labor
  b. Cleansing perineum whenever indicated
  c. Brushing teeth after emesis or during long labor
  d. Washing hands after elimination when confined to bed
5. Encourage frequent change of position and appropriate activity.[23]
  a. When in bed, the woman should avoid supine position or use a hip roll to prevent vena caval compression and subsequent maternal hypotension. [1]
  b. Lateral position may decrease frequency of contraction but increase intensity of contractions.
  c. Ambulation and sitting improve efficiency of uterine contractions, assist fetal descent, and may increase comfort.
6. Provide emotional support and labor coaching in accordance with the mother's training.
7. Utilize nonpharmacologic methods for pain relief, e.g., massage, shower or bath, relaxation methods.
8. Offer pharmacologic analgesia (see Table 6-1 for maternal, fetal, and labor effects of specific drugs) when appropriate.
  a. Analgesia decision must consider the following:
    • Stage and phase of labor
    • Contraction pattern
    • Fetal status
    • Maternal desires
    • Presence of allergies
    • Type of birth setting
    • Availability of equipment and personnel for treatment of untoward effects
  b. Choose appropriate analgesia (Table 6-1).
    • Intravenous medication should be given over two to three contractions at the onset of each contraction to minimize dose to infant.

Table 6-1
Effects of Selected Sedatives and Analgesics Used in Labor [7,19,26]

Classification of Drug	Standard Dose (mg)	Onset (min)	Duration (hr)	Effect on Labor	Maternal Effect	Fetal Newborn Effects
Sedatives						
Barbituates: commonly used in false labor or women with prolonged latent phase although effectiveness for this purpose is questionable						
Pentobarbital (Nembutal)	IM: to 100 IV: 50 PO: to 100	10-15 5 10-15	3-4	Large amounts can decrease uterine activity and prolong labor	CNS depressant: moderate sedation and lethargy; nausea and vomiting	May improve fetal asphyxia in utero[7]; large doses cause respiratory depression and not easily reversible; drowsiness and decreased sucking may occur for 2-4 days
Secobarbital	IM: to 100 IM: to 50 PO: to 100	10-15 5 10-15	3-4	As above	Moderate sedation	
Tranquilizers*						
Promethazine (Phenergan)	IM: 25-50 q4-6 hr IV: 25 q3-4 hr (use with caution)	20 3-5	4-6 2-4	Increase intensity and frequency of contractions	Moderate sedative; relief of anxiety; antiemetic; possible hypotension	May cause delay of onset of repirations and thermostasis problems
Hydroxyzine (Vistaril)	IM:25-50 q 4-6 hr	15-30	4-6	No effect	Relief of anxiety; antiemetic	May cause delay of onset of respirations and thermostasis problems

148

Propiomazine	IM or IV: 20-40 q3 hr (frequently used with meperidine)	3-4	No effect	Relief of anxiety; women may become excited and delirious or excessively sedated	None documented
Narcotic analgesics†					
Meperidine (Demerol)	IM: 50-100 q 3-4 hr IV: 25-50 q 4 hr	2-4 2-3	Uterine inertia in latent phase; no effect on contractions in active phase; may speed dilation due to relaxation	Good analgesia; side effects: dry mouth, nausea and vomiting, hypotension, diaphoresis	Decrease FHR variability 2-30 min after IV dose; respiratory depression if and most reversible before delivery (least effect and most reversible of all narcotics)
Morphine sulphate	IM: 5-10 IV: 3-5 SC: 8-10	1½-2 2-4 4-5	Uterine inertia in latent phase; no effect on contractions in active phase; may speed dilation due to relaxation; may effect more efficient contractions in irritable uterus	Good analgesia; side effects: dry mouth, nausea and vomiting, hypotension, diaphoresis	Respiratory depression if dose within 3 hr of delivery; causes 10 times cases of depression as other narcotics

Table 6-1 continues.

Table 6-1 continued.

Classification of Drug	Standard Dose (mg)	Onset (min)	Duration (hr)	Effect on Labor	Maternal Effect	Fetal Newborn Effects
Nonnarcotic analgesics						
Butorphanol (stadol)	IM: 1-4 q 3-4 hr IV: 0.5-2	10 3-4 2-3		No effect in active phase	Stronger than morphine; side effects: vertigo, nausea, headache, sweating, respiratory depression	Increases incidence of sinusoildal fetal heart rate pattern[10]; less respiratory depression than narcotics
Nalbuphine HCI (Nubain)	IM: 10-20 q 3-4 hr SC: 10-20 IV: 5	10-15 10-15 2-3	3-6 4	No effect in active phase	Subjective: less lethargy and nausea than narcotics	Less respiratory depression than narcotics
Inhalants‡						
Nitrous oxide	30-50% concentration	30-45 sec	3 min	None: initiate 30-40 sec prior to onset of contraction	Good analgesia especially late first stage: side effects: tingling sensation, dizziness or giddiness, increased sensitivity to sound	Possible hypoxia and myocardial depression if greater than 50%

150

Table 6-1 continued.

Nonnarcotic analgesics

Classification of Drug	Standard Dose (mg)	Onset (min)	Duration (hr)	Effect on Labor	Maternal Effect	Fetal Newborn Effects
Butorphanol (stadol)	IM: 1-4 q 3-4 hr IV: 0.5-2	10 3-4 2-3		No effect in active phase	Stronger than morphine; side effects: vertigo, nausea, headache, sweating, respiratory depression	Increases incidence of sinusoidal fetal heart rate pattern[10], less respiratory depression than narcotics
Nalbuphine HCl (Nubain)	IM: 10-20 q 3-4 hr SC: 10-20 IV: 5	10-15 10-15 2-3	3-6 4	No effect in active phase	Subjective: less lethargy and nausea than narcotics	Less respiratory depression than narcotics

Inhalants‡

Classification of Drug	Standard Dose (mg)	Onset (min)	Duration (hr)	Effect on Labor	Maternal Effect	Fetal Newborn Effects
Nitrous oxide	30-50% concentration	30-45 sec	3 min	None: initiate 30-40 sec prior to onset of contraction	Good analgesia especially late first stage: side effects: tingling sensation, dizziness or giddiness, increased sensitivity to sound	Possible hypoxia and myocardial depression if greater than 50%

151

- Inhalational analgesia must be self-administered by the woman. (See Table 6-1 for maximum concentrations.)
- Paracervical analgesia should be given as appropriate to setting and emergency facilities.
- Consult with physician prior to request for conduction analgesia.
9. Continue assessment of labor.
    a. Evaluate uterine contractions for frequency, duration, and intensity by palpation or internal pressure catheter as appropriate.

External tocodynamometers can assess only relative frequency, not qualitative strength of contractions.

---

    b. Perform cervical examinations for dilation, effacement, station, and position, as appropriate to the following:
    - Change in labor pattern
    - Change in maternal affect
    - Rupture of membranes
    - Change in fetal heart rate pattern
    c. Perform amniotomy as appropriate and only if woman is in active labor with an engaged vertex presentation and is a minimum of 4 cm dilated.[17]
    d. Document labor progress; use of modified Friedman labor curve graph is very helpful.
    e. Consult physician for lack of labor progress (dilation or descent) for 2-3 hours in active phase.
B. Ongoing assessment of fetal status
    1. Assessment may be by auscultation or electronic monitoring, externally or internally, continuously or intermittently.
    2. If intermittent, assessment should be every 30 minutes in early labor, and every 15 minutes in active labor, with auscultation through two full contraction cycles.
    3. Observe baseline fetal heart rate (normal, 120-160). With internal monitoring, note presence of both long and short term variability (normal > 5 bpm).

With some newer monitors, long-term variability can be assessed externally fairly accurately.

---

    4. If variability is decreased, apply fetal scalp electrode to confirm.
    5. Note any deceleration or acceleration patterns.
    6. Document above findings appropriately.
    7. Consult with physician if any of the above are not within normal limits.
    8. Attempt to correct abnormal fetal heart status with the following:
        a. Maternal position change.

b. Administration of O_2 via mask or nasal catheter to mother

c. Elimination of a hypertonic contraction pattern by discontinuing oxytocin if being infused

d. Increase in IV fluids

III. Management of stage II

A. Assessment of maternal status

1. Observe for characteristics of stage II (see I, B, 4, a).

2. Instruct the woman when to begin pushing.

   a. After complete dilation

   b. When the woman feels the urge to push (except for the woman with conduction anesthesia who feels no urge)[2]

   c. Pushing prior to complete dilation should be discouraged to prevent cervical edema and lacerations

3. Teach proper bearing-down technique.

   a. Open-glottis pushing is preferred for anatomic and physiologic reasons.[5,27]

   b. Traditional instruction is a sustained Valsalva maneuver.

4. Provide emotional support and direction through constant presence of self or other qualified professional.

5. Assess bladder for overdistention. If present, and woman is unable to void, she may need catheterization.

6. Consult with physician for lack of fetal descent after 1-2 hours of good pushing effort (normal descent is 1 cm/hr).

B. Assessment of fetal status

1. Auscultate fetal heart rate every 5 minutes during and after every contraction.

   a. If using a fetoscope, auscultate during an entire contraction cycle to detect late decelerations.

   b. If electronic monitoring is being used, use continuously until delivery.

2. Observe perineum for presence of meconium-stained fluid (see Section V, F).

3. Consult physician for late decelerations, moderate to severe variable deceleration, decreased variability, or tachycardia.

4. If sudden, unresponsive bradycardia is noted, notify physician stat and prepare for delivery.

IV. Delivery management

A. General policies

1. Spontaneous vaginal delivery of a single fetus in the vertex presentation may be performed by a nonphysician provider, e.g., certified nurse-midwife, with or without direct supervision of a physician.

2. Some settings may provide for practitioner and physician comanagement of the following:

    a. Spontaneous vaginal delivery of a twin gestation presenting vertex-vertex

    b. Spontaneous vaginal delivery of a single fetus in breech presentation

  3. If any delivery complication or difficulty is suspected, e.g., shoulder dystocia, the following should be done:

    a. Woman should be transferred to a hospital setting if in an out-of-hospital birth site.

    b. Practitioner should request that an obstetrician and/or pediatrician be available as appropriate.

B. Management of delivery

  1. Prepare for delivery when head is distending perineum in primigravida and when cervix is dilated 8-10 cm in multipara.

  2. Ensure a quiet and safe environment for the delivery.

  3. Allow woman to choose delivery position most comfortable for her unless intervening variable is present.[24]

    a. Semisitting position: may not be appropriate with large infant and a delivery bed that does not allow downward traction for shoulders

    b. Squatting position

    c. Side-lying or lateral position

    d. Hands and knees position

    e. Supine modified lithotomy position: avoid vena cava compression with a hip roll

  4. Cleaning perineum with an antiseptic solution is optional; if it is done, be aware of woman's allergy status.

  5. Provide adequate perineal anesthesia as appropriate.

    a. Local infiltration: use lidocaine HCl (Xylocaine) 1 percent in 10-ml divided dose (not to exceed 50 ml).

    b. Pudendal block: use lidocaine HCl (Xylocaine) 1 percent in a dose of 10-ml per side (not to exceed 50 ml).

    c. Consult for other anesthesia techniques (epidural, spinal, saddle block) administered by physician or nurse anesthetist.

  6. Institute appropriate measures to avoid perineal lacerations or episiotomy, as follows:

    a. Apply moist heat to perineum.

    b. Encourage slow distension of perineum.

    c. Encourage slow, controlled delivery, keeping vertex flexed.

    d. Attempt delivery between contractions.

  7. Perform midline episiotomy[4] if indicated, as follows:

    a. To avoid uncontrolled tears, including extension into rectum

    b. To counter the arrest of progress by a resistant perineum

    c. For fetal indications: large infant, occiput posterior position, abnormal presentation, fetal distress

    d. Per maternal request

  8. Deliver infant in as gentle and nontraumatic a manner as possible.

    a. If meconium has been noted, suction mouth and nasopharynx with De-

Lee trap or mechanical suction on perineum prior to delivery of shoulders.
9. If shoulder dystocia is encountered, follow these steps [21]:
   a. Ask for qualified assistance stat.
   b. Cut or extend episiotomy.
   c. Deliver shoulders in oblique position before external rotation occurs, avoiding excessive traction.
   d. Have assistant apply suprapubic pressure as mother bears down with hyperflexed hips, or deliver posterior shoulder by inserting hand along sacrum, grasping an arm, and drawing it across chest of fetus into the vagina.
10. Provide warm environment and position conducive to mucus draining for infant: directly on mother's abdomen is best unless contraindicated, e.g., if there is a need to visualize vocal cords because meconium is present, or if there is a depressed infant.
C. Management of third stage
   1. Collect cord bloods for blood type and Rh and Venereal Disease Research Laboratories (VDRL) or other infectious disease screening as appropriate.
   2. Deliver placenta, membranes, and cord, checking for the following:
      a. Presence of three cord vessels
      b. Completeness of membranes and cotyledons
      c. Any abnormalities
   3. If placenta has not delivered within 30 minutes, consult physician. If bleeding is not excessive, the physician may authorize further waiting. Transfer to hospital may be necessary if in an out-of-hospital birth setting. A semisitting or squatting position to facilitate the force of gravity may be helpful.
   4. If the placenta is not delivered, and bleeding is excessive, do the following:
      a. Ask for assistance.
      b. Attempt manual removal of the placenta.
      c. Prepare for surgical intervention and notify physician stat if placenta is adherent.
      d. Increase IV fluids or start IV stat.
   5. If placenta or membranes are not intact, perform manual exploration of the uterus as appropriate to practice setting or request procedure be done by physician.
   6. Massage uterine fundus after delivery of placenta until firm and well contracted.
   7. Possibly administer oxytocic drugs after placenta is delivered.
      a. Indications for oxytocic use are the following:
         • Uterus does not contract with massage.
         • There is an increased risk of postpartum hemorrhage due to the following:
           — Overdistended uterus

- High parity
- History of previous postpartum hemorrhage
- Prolonged labor
- Precipitous labor/delivery
- Use of oxytocin during labor

 b. Usual oxytocic drugs and doses are as follows:

- Ten units of oxytocin (Pitocin) IM, or
- Ten units of oxytocin in 500 ml of intravenous fluid infused at 125 ml/hr (not to exceed 300 ml/hr), or
- Methylergonovine (Methergine) or ergonovine maleate (Ergotrate), 0.2 mg IM if blood pressure (BP) not above 130/80

 c. In some settings, oxytocics are administered with delivery of the anterior shoulder. This technique should be used with caution because of the possibility of unsuspected twins and cervical spasm causing trapping of the placenta.[15]

8. Perform bimanual compression in the presence of uterine atony unresponsive to drugs and fundal massage. Consult with physician if bleeding continues.
9. Inspect the vagina, cervix, and perineum for evidence of bleeding and/or lacerations.
10. Repair episiotomy or any second degree lacerations (done by appropriate personnel).
11. Repair third or fourth degree lacerations or cervical lacerations with medical supervision as appropriate to level of competence, role in the setting, and state regulations.
12. Perform a rectal exam to identify occult fourth-degree laceration and assess integrity of sphincter and/or presence of suture in the rectum.
13. Clean perineum and provide ice pack to decrease edema.
14. Explain to parents extent of any lacerations, length of time before sutures dissolve, and any special care measures.
15. Assess total amount of blood loss.
16. Document delivery and third-stage management completely, especially noting any problems such as shoulder dystocia or uterine atony and newborn's transition.
17. Sign or make provisions for proper completion of birth certificate and submission to appropriate vital statistics agency.

D. Management of the immediate newborn transition

1. Perform nasal/oral suction via bulb syringe with the delivery of the head (see Section III, B, 3, h, and V, F if meconium present).
2. Pediatrician or qualified person in neonatal resuscitation should be present at birth if fetal distress is present or anticipated.
3. Promote establishment of respirations and patent airway after birth with stimulation by drying infant, and performing postural drainage and bulb suctioning as necessary.

4. Perform initial assessment of the newborn and assign Apgar scores at 1 and 5 minutes.
5. Promote early infant-parent contact especially skin-to-skin contact.
6. Observe newborn for signs of difficulties making fetal-to-newborn transition, including dusky color, grunting, and apnea.
7. Order or apply eye prophylaxis to newborn. Use of erythromycin ointment is considered preferable to cover both *Neisseria gonorrhea* and *chlamydia*.
8. Order or give vitamin K, 1 mg IM, to promote clotting.

E. Management of the immediate postpartum period
1. Provide a clean, comfortable, quiet environment for the mother.
2. Compliment mother, family, and/or friends on their efforts.
3. Assess and record uterine contractility, fundal height, estimated blood loss, and pulse and blood pressure every 15 minutes for a minimum of 1 hour, until stable, or per protocols. Take temperature once.
4. Encourage successful breast-feeding (if selected by mother) by placing baby to breast as soon after delivery as possible and giving basic instructions in breast-feeding technique.
5. Instruct bottle-feeding mother in measures to minimize breast engorgement.
6. Observe parent-infant interaction and note any possible stressors.
7. Encourage early voiding to avoid bladder distension and possible uterine atony. (See Chapter 7, Section II, C).
8. Provide nourishing meal to mother and encourage intake of fluids.
9. If bleeding is excessive, do the following:
   a. Check contractility of uterus and massage if boggy. Give oxytocic drugs as approporiate.
   b. Check height and placement of fundus. If misplaced due to large bladder, ensure adequate voiding or catheterize if necessary.
   c. Massage fundus, guarding the lower uterine segment above the symphysis, to expel any clots.
   d. Check vagina and perineum for unrepaired lacerations if bleeding is bright red in color.
   e. Consult with physician if bleeding continues after above measures or if vital signs are abnormal.

V. Special considerations

A. Failure to progress in active labor[20]
1. Determine failure to progress by arrest of dilation (less than 1 cm/hr in primigravida and 1.5 cm/hr in multigravida) or arrest of fetal descent for 2 hours.
2. Evaluate fetus for the following:
   a. Size: macrosomia

    b. Conditions preventing flexion, i.e., anomalies of neck or hydrocephalus

    c. Position (see Section IV, J)

    d. Asynclitism

  3. Reevaluate pelvis: measure the following:

    a. Inlet by diagonal conjugate (more than 12.5 adequate for average baby).

    b. Mid-pelvis by assessing sidewalls and ischial spines: converging sidewalls and prominent spines may indicate contracted mid-pelvis

    c. Outlet
- Subpubic arch (less than 90 degrees narrow)
- Diameter of ischial tuberosities (less than 8 cm narrow).

  4. Evaluate uterine contractions for frequency, intensity, and duration.

  5. Consult with physician regarding above findings.

    a. If absolute cephalopelvic disproportion is suspected, transfer to physician. Inform couple of reason for transfer.

    b. If a hypotonic labor is suspected, do the following:
- Consider change of woman's activity to increase contractions.
- Treat maternal anxiety if present since anxiety causes release of catecholamines, which can cause uterine dysfunction.[14]
- Ensure adequate hydration.
- Consider intrauterine contraction monitoring to confirm hypotonic labor pattern and/or oxytocin augmentation, as necessary.

B. Fever greater than 100.4° F or 38° C

  1. History

    a. Fever prior to labor

    b. Recent exposure to infectious disease or viral syndrome

    c. Complaints of upper respiratory infection

    d. Symptoms of gastrointestinal or genitourinary infection

    e. Generalized feelings of malaise

    f. Labor status and status of membranes

    g. Previous risk factors: e.g., pyelonephritis during pregnancy.

    h. Length of rupture of membranes

  2. Physical exam: to rule out site of infection other than uterus

  3. Laboratory studies

    a. Obtain usual complete blood count (CBC) and urinalysis.

    b. Order a urine culture and sensitivities.

    c. Perform blood cultures as indicated.

    d. Obtain cervical cultures as indicated.

  4. Management and teaching

    a. Consult with physician regarding management plan.

    b. If etiology known, treat appropriately and document in chart.

    c. If low grade fever without obvious etiology, hydrate the woman.

    d. Check temperature every hour.

    e. Monitor fetus closely for fetal tachycardia and loss of fetal heart rate (FHR) variability.

f. If delivery is estimated to occur in 1-2 hours, try to withhold antibiotics so cultures of the baby will not be affected.

g. At time of delivery, notify the pediatrician of the mother's status.

h. Obtain placental cultures post-delivery.

i. In an out-of-hospital birth setting, woman should be transferred to a hospital for intravenous antibiotics.

j. Prepare mother for at least 2-day hospital stay if endometritis is the diagnosis.

k. Prepare the parents for the kind of fever workup their pediatrician prefers.

C. Gestational diabetes: non-insulin dependent patients

In some settings, nonphysician providers may assume intrapartum management of gestational diabetics who are in good control. However, these women are not candidates for out-of-hospital births.

---

1. History
   a. Review chart for recent blood sugar levels and make sure they are within normal limits.
   b. Review chart for any additional risk factors:
      • Suspicion of macrosomic infant
      • Concern or diagnosis of intrauterine growth retardation
      • Symptoms of pregnancy-induced hypertension (PIH)
   c. Confirm gestational age with patient and chart review. Concern that infant is less than 37 weeks or greater than 41 weeks gestation should result in physician consult.
   d. Ask the woman time and quantity of her last meal.
2. Physical exam: routinely conducted physical with particular attention to abdominal exam to ascertain macrosomia and/or polyhydramnios
3. Laboratory studies: the usual (see Section I, C), with the addition of a random blood sugar on admission
4. Management and teaching
   a. Intravenous infusion is not mandatory except in the presence of macrosomia or other risk factors.
   b. If intravenous infusion is used, 5 percent dextrose with lactated Ringer's should be used, not to exceed 100 ml/hr.
   c. If an intravenous bolus is required, as for hydration or conduction anesthesia, a normal saline solution should be used.
   d. Continuous fetal monitoring is mandatory.

D. Herpes type II: history with negative cultures
1. History
   a. Review chart or ask woman the date of last outbreak of lesions.

      b. Ascertain if recent herpes culture is negative.

      c. Question woman carefully about current presence of lesions or sensations of burning or itching at site of usual outbreaks.

      d. Elicit labor status and status of membranes.

  2. Physical exam

      a. Carefully examine external genitalia for lesions.

      b. Perform speculum exam to visualize any lesions on vaginal walls or cervix.

      c. If a possible herpetic lesion is visualized, scrape lesion for lab studies.

  3. Laboratory studies

      a. Prepare a slide for Tzanck smear or Gram stain.

      b. Obtain herpes culture if appropriate.

  4. Management and teaching

      a. If no lesions are visualized:

        • Reassure woman of negative exam.

        • Proceed with usual labor management except utilize amniotomy and fetal scalp electrode only if indicated as further precaution for undetected incipient infection.

      b. If a lesion is visualized:

        • Consult with physician for immediate cesarean section

        • Discuss management plan with parents and prepare them for cesarean section.

E. Magnesium sulphate ($MgSO_4$) infusion

  1. History (see Section V, H)

  2. Physical exam

      a. Obtain baseline vital signs and FHR pattern.

      b. Elicit deep tendon reflexes and presence of clonus and document for baseline.

      c. Assess amount and location of edema if present.

  3. Laboratory studies

      a. Perform baseline studies (see Section V, H).

      b. Draw magnesium levels every 6-8 hours to ascertain therapeutic blood level (4-6 mEq/ml is therapeutic).

  4. Management and teaching

      a. Consult with physician regarding comanagement per protocol.

      b. Administer 4-6 g loading dose of $MgSO_4$ over 15-20 minutes.

      c. Inform mother she may experience flushing, nausea, and/or vomiting.

      d. Initiate maintenance dose of $MgSO_4$ per physician order (usually 2-2.5 g/hr) using infusion pump.

      e. Check mother's blood pressure, respirations, intake and output (may use indwelling catheter), and reflexes hourly.

      f. Continuously monitor fetal heart rate.

      g. Consult with physician:

        • If there are depressed respirations (less than 10-14/min)

        • If there are absent or increased reflexes

- If there is decreased urine output (less than 30 ml/hr or 100 ml/4 hr).

    h. Discontinue maintenance dose after 24 hours postpartum if vital signs are normal, symptoms of PIH are absent, and physician approval has been obtained.

    i. Consult physician if postpartum exam is not within normal limits.

F. Meconium-stained amniotic fluid

1. History

    a. Elicit from mother time of rupture of membranes and color of fluid.

    b. Review chart for risk factors for fetal distress:

    - Suspicion of intrauterine growth retardation
    - History of drug abuse
    - Presence of hypertension
    - Post dates

2. Physical exam

    a. Observe for gross rupture of meconium fluid on perineum, pad, or underwear.

    b. Observe for meconium-stained fluid on sterile speculum exam.

    c. Meconium fluid is usually rated as follows:

    - Light or + 1: fluid thin and watery with greenish color
    - Moderate or + 2: thicker green fluid but still liquid
    - Heavy or + 3: fluid like pea soup—very thick, with particulate matter

    d. Breech presentations will normally have meconium present, but fetal distress should always be considered.

3. Management and teaching

    a. Women with moderate or heavy meconium-stained fluid in an out-of-hospital birth setting should be transferred to a hospital.

    b. Continuous fetal monitoring (internal or external) is recommended since presence of meconium may be a sign of fetal distress.

    c. Consult with physician if signs of fetal distress are noted.

    d. Make sure personnel trained in neonatal intubation and resuscitation are present at birth.

    e. Suction mouth and nasopoharyanyx with DeLee trap or mechanical suction with delivery of the head prior to delivery of the shoulders.

    f. Cut cord promptly so assessment of presence of meconium below the vocal cords can be made quickly.

    g. Discuss with parents the possible implications, if any, at time meconium is noted.

    h. Obtain mother's cooperation at delivery to allow thorough suctioning on the perineum through prior discussion of importance of not pushing after delivery of head.

G. Oxytocin augmentation or induction

1. History

    a. If physician has ordered oxytocin for induction, confirm with physician that all available data confirm gestational age. The patient must meet the following criteria[3]:

- Well-established ovulation date determined by one of the following:
  — Regular menstrual history prior to LMP
  — Basal body temperature chart
  — Clomiphene induction of ovulation
  — Artificial insemination
- Early exam by 14th week with size equal to dates
- Fetal heart tones heard with fetoscope by 20th week of pregnancy
- Fetal weight estimated as 6 pounds or more
- Bishop score of 9 or more (Table 6-2).

b. If gestational age is in doubt, refer to physician for further evaluation.
c. Review history and chart to assure mother does not have any of the following:
   - Contraindications
     — Shoulder presentation
     — Previous classical cesarean section
     — Fetal distress
     — Placenta praevia
   - Relative contraindications
     — Previous low transverse cesarean section
     — Breech presentation
     — Overdistended uterus, i.e., multiple gestation polyhydramnios, multiparity > 5
     — Suspected cephalo-pelvic disproportion (CPD)
     — Inability to monitor FHR during labor

2. Physical exam
   a. Evaluate present contraction pattern by electronic monitor whenever possible. (Hypertonic uterine activity is a contraindication.)
   b. Perform vaginal exam for the following:
      - Dilation and effacement
      - Station and presentation
      - Consistency and position of cervix
      - Status of membranes

Table 6-2
Bishop Score

Factor	0	1	2	3
Dilation(cm)	0	1-2	3-4	5-6
Effacement (%)	0-30	40-50	60-70	80
Station*	-3	-2	-1 or 0	+1 or +2
Consistency	Firm	Medium	Soft	
Position	Posterior	Midline	Anterior	

*Station: centimeters above (-) or below (+) level of ischial spines of bony pelvis.

    c. Determine Bishop score (Table 6-2)
3. Management and teaching[18]
    a. If augmentation is to be undertaken, consult with physician to report physical findings and labor status and to obtain order for oxytocin augmentation.
    b. Continuous uterine and fetal monitoring must be utilized.
    c. Begin infusion of oxytocin at 0.5-1 mU/min IV. (Utilize a mechanical constant infusion pump to ensure accurate dosage and delivery rate.)
    d. A trained professional should always be in attendance when oxytocin is being infused.
    e. Increase oxytocin in 2 mU/min increments every 20 minutes (or per protocol) until adequate contractions are achieved (every 3-4 minutes; 50-60-second duration).
    f. Decrease oxytocin as indicated by frequency or duration of contraction pattern.
    g. Consult with physician if 20-mU/min dose is reached without adequate contractions.
    h. Document dose, contraction pattern, and fetal status hourly.
    i. Discontinue oxytocin infusion if the following occurs:
      • Tetanic or prolonged contractions (> 2 minutes)
      • Unusual vaginal bleeding
      • Mother complains of severe abdominal pain in absence of a contraction
      • Fetal distress noted by an abnormal FHR pattern
    j. If fetal distress is noted, do the following:
      • Turn off oxytocin
      • Turn woman on her left side
      • Administer oxygen via mask or nasal prongs
      • Notify physician
      • Increase IV fluids
      • Document all procedures and effects
    k. Tetanic contractions should resolve within minutes of discontinuing infusion since half-life of oxytocin is 1-3 minutes.
H. Mild pregnancy-induced hypertension: an increase of 30 mm Hg systolic or 15 mm Hg diastolic over baseline readings or greater than 140/90 with either proteinuria or edema

---

Women who have severe PIH by the following criteria must be immediately referred to a physician[22]

1. BP > 160 systolic or > 110 diastolic.
2. Proteinuria > 5 gm/24 hours (3+ or 4+ qualitative)
3. Oliguria (< 500 ml/24 hours)
4. Cerebral or visual disturbances
5. Epigastric pain
6. Pulmonary edema

1. History
    a. Presence of headaches: severity, duration, and location
    b. Presence of blurred vision or spots in front of eyes
    c. Complaints of abdominal pain, referred shoulder pain, or feeling of persistent pressure in mid-sternum.
    d. Edema presence: location and duration
    e. Signs and symptoms of labor
2. Review prenatal record
    a. Risk factors associated with PIH: adolescent or > 40, primigravida, low socioeconomic status, previous history of hypertension, diabetes
    b. Baseline BP readings and any elevations
    c. Previous proteinuria and edema
    d. Baseline reflexes
3. Physical exam
    a. Obtain blood pressure with patient lying on left side.
    b. Perform fundoscopic exam for presence of arterial-venous (A-V) nicking.
    c. Palpate abdomen (right upper quadrant) for hepatic tenderness.
    d. Assess location and amount of edema.
    e. Elicit deep tendon reflexes and note presence of clonus.
4. Laboratory studies
    a. Obtain CBC and platelet count.
    b. Check urine for proteinuria; if protein present, obtain a catheterized specimen to rule out contamination.
    c. Monitor kidney function with blood for urea nitrogen, uric acid, and creatinine.
    d. Assess liver function, including SGOT and SGPT.
5. Management: consult physician regarding findings and decide if collaborative management or transfer to physician care is appropriate

I. Rupture of membranes: term
1. History
    a. Time of onset of vaginal leaking
    b. Amount and color of fluid
    c. Presence or absence of uterine contractions
    d. Presence, color, and amount of bleeding
    e. History of herpes type II.
2. Physical exam
    a. Perform a sterile speculum examination to observe for pooling of fluid and to obtain samples for nitrazine and fern tests. Observe carefully for lesions and obtain cultures or smears as appropriate.
    b. Perform a vaginal exam at discretion of the practitioner based on management plan and labor status.
    c. Palpate abdomen for signs of tenderness possibly indicative of chorioamnionitis.
    d. Note maternal temperature to rule out infection.

e. Note fetal heart rate pattern; fetal tachycardia may be indicative of chorioamnionitis.

3. Laboratory studies
   a. Perform nitrazine test: dark blue color is probably indicative of amniotic fluid. Note that blood and cervical secretions may also turn nitrazine blue.
   b. Examine slides with dried fluid microscopically for presence of ferning or arborization pattern.
   c. Obtain CBC count for baseline.
   d. Consult with physician regarding need to obtain amniotic fluid, via amniocentesis or vaginal pool collection, for lung maturation studies if gestational age is questionable.

4. Conservative management[12]

Women managed this way are at increased risk of infection that may affect the baby but they are at less risk of a failed induction in the presence of an unfavorable cervix, which might result in a cesarean section.

---

a. Performance of a vaginal exam is controversial. Unless otherwise indicated, a cervical exam is not done. (Spontaneous labor will occur in a significant number of women with spontaneous rupture of membranes [SROM].)
b. Nontraditional treatment to encourage onset of labor in the term mother may include the following:
   • Castor oil: 60 ml orally one time or 30 ml every hour x 3[8]
   • Phosphate or soap-sud enema
c. The following women are good candidates for this management:
   • Those with term gestation with unfavorable cervix, e.g., long and closed
   • Those not infected and able to understand danger signs of infection and who can comply with close follow-up
   • Those who choose this management
d. Prior to sending the woman home, do the following:
   • Make sure no signs or symptoms of uterine infection are present.
   • Ensure good fetal status, e.g., reactive nonstress test.
   • Perform ultrasound profile for fetal status and the presence of adequate amniotic fluid.
   • Review risks and benefits with the woman and document your instructions and woman's understanding of them.
e. Instruct the woman to do the following:
   • Monitor her temperature three times a day and notify provider if > 100° F.
   • Notify provider if fluid becomes profuse, foul smelling, purulent, or green in color.

- Palpate abdomen twice daily for tenderness and notify provider if present.
- Notify provider if fetal movement is decreased.
- Maintain pelvic rest and avoid tub baths.
- Return for follow-up; daily visits at term for fetal heart rate are ideal (frequently the first sign of uterine infection is fetal tachycardia).
5. Aggressive management

The goal of this management is to deliver the baby less than 24 hours after rupture of membranes to decrease risk of infection to infant.

---

a. Consult with physician regarding oxytocin induction/augmentation or nipple stimulation to obtain an adequate contraction pattern.
b. Some providers may wait 6-12 hours after SROM for spontaneous onset of labor before instituting oxytocin. Use of prostaglandin gel during this time, although in experimental stage, may become an important adjunct to management.[13]
c. Vaginal exams should be kept to a minimum.
d. Repeat CBC every 12 hours to monitor possible infection.
e. Pediatrician should be notified at delivery if woman is febrile or if membranes have been ruptured more than 24 hours.
f. Women with a recent positive herpes culture or an active lesion require immediate physician consult.

J. Unusual presentations or positions[20]
1. Occiput posterior position
   a. Subjective information: woman may experience a great deal of low back pain
   b. Diagnosis:
      - Note irregularly shaped abdomen, i.e., indentation at or below umbilicus, sometimes confused with a full bladder.
      - There should be easy palpation of small parts abdominally.
      - Perform palpation of posterior fontanelle posteriorly on vaginal exam.
   c. Management and teaching
      - Provide counter-pressure on low back or use heat or cold for pain relief.
      - Encourage lateral position or hands and knees position with pelvic rocking motion to assist with rotation to anterior position.
      - During second stage, possibly attempt manual rotation with maternal bearing-down effort.
      - Anticipate a longer second stage.
      - Consult with physician for arrest of descent.
2. Face presentation
   a. Diagnosis: by vaginal palpation of facial features; note position of mentum
   b. Management and teaching

- Allow time for mentum posterior to rotate anteriorly.
- This presentation may not meet criteria for an out-of-hospital birth.
- Consult with physician once diagnosis is made and especially if mentum is persistently posterior in late first stage. Transfer the woman to hospital if in out-of-hospital birth setting.
- Prepare the woman for an operative delivery.

3. Brow presentation
   a. Diagnosis
      - Abdominal palpation of the cephalic prominence is on same side as back.
      - There is easy palpation of the anterior fontanelle and supraorbital ridges on vaginal exam.
   b. Management and teaching
      - Allow time for brow to convert to an occiput or face presentation if unengaged.
      - If brow presentation is well engaged, consult with physician and prepare patient for an operative or spontaneous delivery (e.g., small baby with large pelvis).
      - If spontaneous delivery, anticipate the need for a generous episiotomy to allow the passage of a large head diameter.

VI. Guidelines for intrapartum management in alternative settings

A. Factors at the onset of labor that would exclude a woman from delivery in an out-of-hospital delivery site[16] include the following:
   1. Onset of labor before 37 weeks gestation or after 42 weeks
   2. Prolonged rupture of membranes (institutional criteria or length of rupture will vary)
   3. Nonvertex presentation or multiple gestation
   4. Estimated fetal weight < 2500 g or > 4000 g
   5. Evidence of fetal distress, e.g., abnormal heart rate pattern or meconium staining greater than + 1
   6. Maternal vital signs that deviate from normal (e.g., fever, hypertension)
   7. Abnormal vaginal bleeding
B. Factors that develop during labor and/or following delivery that dictate transfer of mother to an in-hospital setting include the following:
   1. Prolapsed cord
   2. Placental abruption
   3. Failure to progress in labor
      a. First stage: protracted active phase or secondary arrest of dilation
      b. Second stage: more than 2 hours without progress in descent
      c. Third stage: more than 1 hour without delivery of placenta
   4. Soft-tissue problems, e.g., severe vulvar varicosities, marked edema of cervix

5. Deviation of maternal or fetal vital signs from the normal
6. Inability of the mother to maintain sufficient control to cooperate fully in the delivery process without pharmacologic analgesia
7. Evidence of meconium in previously clear amniotic fluid
8. Third- or fourth-degree vaginal or cervical lacerations
9. Blood loss preceding or following delivery that exceeds normal expectation
   a. Minimum standard is to consult with physician.
   b. Transfer is dependent on maternal status or degree of control of bleeding.
10. Any condition requiring manual exploration of the uterus
11. Development of other severe medical-surgical problems
12. Evidence of active infectious process
13. Any condition requiring postpartum observation beyond 6-12 hours (dependent on policy of setting)
C. Factors that develop after delivery that dictate transfer of the infant to an in-hospital setting include the following:
   1. Apgar score less than 7 at 5 minutes
   2. Signs of pre- or postmaturity
   3. Evidence of any respiratory instability
   4. Jaundice at birth
   5. Persistent hypothermia
   6. Exaggerated tremors
   7. Major congenital anomaly
   8. Any condition requiring more than 6-12 hours of observation postdelivery (dependent on policy of setting)

REFERENCES

1. Abitol M: Supine position in labor and associated fetal heart rate changes. Obstet Gynec 65(4):481-486, 1985
2. Beynon C: The normal second stage of labour. J Obstet Gynecol Br Emp 64:815-820, 1957
3. Bowes W: Clinical aspects of normal labor and abnormal labor, in Creasy R, Resnik R, (eds): Maternal-Fetal Medicine. Philadelphia, Saunders, 1984
4. Bromberg M: Presumptive maternal benefits of routine episiotomy—A literature review. J Nurse-Midwifery 31(3):121-127, 1986
5. Caldeyro-Barcia R, Giussi G, Storch E, et al: The bearing-down effects on fetal heart rate, oxygenation, and acid-base balance. J Perinat Med 9(1):63-67, 1981
6. Carmen S: Neonatal hypoglycemia in response to maternal glucose infusion during delivery. JOG Nurs, 15(4):319-323, 1986
7. Cosmi E: Obstetric Anesthesia and Perinatology. New York, Appleton-Century-Crofts, 1981

8. Davis L: The use of castor oil to stimulate labor in patients with premature rupture of membranes. J Nurse-Midwifery 29(6):366-370, 1984

9. Gregory G, Gooding C, Phibbs R, et al: Meconium aspiration in infants—A prospective study. J Pediatr, 85(6):848-852, 1974

10. Hatjis C, Meis P: Sinusoidal fetal heart rate pattern associated with butorphenol administration. Obstet Gynecol 67(3):377, 1986

11. Hazle N: Hydration in labor: Is routine intravenous hydration necessary? J Nurse-Midwifery 31(4):171-176, 1986

12. Kappy K, et al: Premature rupture of the membranes at term. J Reprod Med 27(1): 29-33, 1982

13. Laube D, Laube D, Zlatnik F, Pitkin R: Preinduction cervical ripening with prostaglandin E2 intracervical gel. Obstet Gynecol 68(1):54-57, 1986

14. Lederman R, Lederman E, Work B, et al: The relationship of maternal anxiety, plasma catecholamines, and plasma cortisol to progress of labor. Am J Obstet Gynecol 132(5):495-500, 1978

15. Long P: Management of the third stage of labor: A review. J Nurse-Midwifery 31(3):135-140, 1986

16. Lubic R: Evaluation of an out-of-hospital maternity center for low-risk patients in Aiken L (ed): Health Policy and Nursing Practice. New York, McGraw-Hill, 1980

17. Lynaugh K: The effects of early elective amniotomy on the length of labor and the condition of the fetus. J Nurse-Midwifery 25(4):3-9, 1980

18. Marshall C: The art of induction/augmentation of labor. JOGN Nurs 14(1):22-28, 1985

19. Myles M: Textbook for Midwives. Edinburgh:, Churchill Livingstone, 1985

20. Oxorn H: Human Labor and Birth. (ed 5). Norwalk, CT, Appleton-Century-Crofts, 1986

21. Resnik R: Management of shoulder dystocia. Clin Obstet Gynecol 23(2):559-564, 1980

22. Roberts J: Pregnancy-related hypertension, in Creasy R, Resnik R (eds): Maternal-Fetal Medicine. Philadelphia, Saunders, 1984

23. Roberts J, Mendez-Bauer G, Wodell D: The effects of maternal position on uterine contractility and efficiency. Birth 10(4):243-249, 1983

24. Roberts J, VanLier D: Debate: Which position for the second stage? Childbirth Educator 3:33-41, 1984

25. Varney H: Nurse-Midwifery. Boston, Blackwell Scientific, 1980

26. Vestal K, McKenzie C: High Risk Perinatal Nursing. Philadelphia, Saunders, 1983

27. Yeates D, Roberts J: A comparison of two bearing-down techniques during the second stage of labor. J Nurse-Midwifery 29(1):3-11, 1984

Chapter 7

Postpartum Management

Mary Ann Rhode

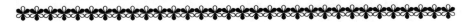

I. Routine postpartum management[59,66]

A. Purpose of daily postpartum visits
   1. Maintain continuity of care
   2. Evaluate postpartum physical and emotional condition of the mother and screen for complications.[2,43,61]
   3. Encourage mother and father, if present, to discuss birth experience.[2,43,61]
   4. Assess condition of infant either by examining infant or obtaining information from nursery. Make sure mother is aware of and understands infant's condition.
   5. Evaluate mother's educational needs and develop a plan to meet those needs.
   6. Provide praise and encouragement.
   7. Teach self-assessment skills.
   8. Enhance parental problem-solving abilities and self-esteem.
   9. Assess support systems—family, social, and professional—adequate or inadequate, positive or negative.
   10. Evaluate parent-child interaction and promote positive family integration.
   11. Initiate referrals to other health care providers or agencies as indicated.
   12. Develop a plan for discharge.
B. Chart review
   1. Review mother's medical record including previous orders and progress notes.
   2. Obtain or review previous temperature, blood pressure, and pulse readings.
   3. Review laboratory reports.
C. History: obtain mother's impression of her physical condition and elicit problems relating to the following:
   1. Appetite
   2. Level of fatigue
   3. Bowel and bladder function
   4. Condition of breasts and nipples

171

     5. Presence or absence of afterpains
     6. Level of perineal discomfort
     7. Amount and type of lochia, presence or absence of clots, odor
     8. Success or problems with infant feeding
D. Physical exam[69]
     1. Examine breasts for the following:
        a. Presence or absence of bra
        b. Adequacy of support of breasts
        c. Size and shape, tissue turgor (soft, firm, hard)
        d. Skin color and tension
        e. Presence or absence of striae
        f. Size and tension of areola
        g. Condition of nipple including tissue integrity
        h. Amount and color of colostrum for breast-feeding mothers
     2. Auscultate lung fields. This portion of exam is not routinely performed in some settings. Fever, cough, congestion, or other respiratory system symptoms would necessitate its inclusion. Postoperative mothers must have their lung fields auscultated with further evaluation as necessary.
     3. Assess lochia for the following:
        a. Color
        b. Amount
        c. Odor
        d. Presence or absence of clots and their number and size (lochia should be assessed prior to palpation of fundus to most accurately assess flow)
     4. Examine uterine fundus for the following:
        a. Size
        b. Shape
        c. Consistency
        d. Location in relation to midline of abdomen
        e. Height in relation to umbilicus
     5. Assess bladder[41]
        a. Inspect for distended bladder.
        b. Palpate suprapubic area to determine fullness of bladder.
     6. Assess abdominal wall and musculature for the following:
        a. Tone
        b. Presence or absence of striae, scars, and linea nigra
        c. Diastasis of abdominal recti muscles: length, width, and depth (examination for separation may be unreliable before 3 days postpartum due to slackness of abdominal muscles[49])
        d. Bowel sounds in mothers who have had tubal ligations or cesarean sections
     7. Examine perineum and anal area. Proper positioning and lighting is essential. Examine for the following:
        a. Redness: presence or absence and extent
        b. Edema: presence or absence and extent

      c. Ecchymosis: presence or absence and extent

      d. Discharge: amount, character, and odor

      e. Approximation of suture line if episiotomy or lacerations are present

      f. Induration: presence or absence, and extent

      g. Hematoma: presence or absence, location, and size

      h. Hemorrhoids: presence or absence, size, condition, and number

      i. Varicosities

      j. A numerical score or REEDA (for redness, edema, ecchymosis, discharge, approximation) score, for evaluation of postpartum perineal healing may be obtained. (REEDA scores are particularly useful for research purposes[12] [Table 7-1]).

   8. Examine legs for the following:

      a. Redness

      b. Warmth

      c. Tenderness

      d. Varicosities

      e. Edema

      f. Homan's sign

      g. Deep tendon reflexes (if mother has a hypertensive disorder of pregnancy or is on magnesium sulfate therapy)

E. Assess postpartum psychological status[40]

   1. Fatigue or energy level

   2. Reaction to labor and delivery experience

   3. Mood or affect

   4. Self esteem and confidence level

   5. Evidence of maternal role behaviors

      a. Degree of dependence or independence

      b. Interest in infant

      c. Caretaking activity

   6. Problem-solving abilities

   7. Presence and quality of available emotional support

   8. Educational level

   9. Amount of previous experience caring for infants[11]

F. Assess parent-infant interaction

   1. Specific behaviors indicative of the quality of the parent-infant interaction should be observed and documented in the mother's medical record.

   2. Assessment may be qualitative or quantitative. (Several assessment tools are available in the nursing literature if a checklist approach to observation is desired.[23,53,55])

   3. Note behaviors commonly considered to be important to the developing interaction[6,8,40]:

      a. Nature and amount of touching

      b. Nature and amount of eye-to-eye contact

      c. Type and amount of vocal communication

      d. Ability of mother to find pleasure in her infant and infant care activities

Table 7-1
REEDA Scale

Points	Redness	Edema	Ecchymosis	Discharge	Approximation
0	None	None	None	None	Closed
1	Within 0.25 cm of incision bilaterally	Perineal, less than 1 cm from incision	Less than 1 cm from incision	Serum	Skin separation of 3 mm or less
2	Within 0.5 cm of incision bilaterally	Perineal and/or vulvar, 1-2 cm from incision	Between 1 and 2 cm from incision	Serosanguinous	Skin and subcutaneous fat separation
3	Beyond 0.5 cm of incision bilaterally	Perineal and/or vulvar, greater than 2 cm from incision	Greater than 2 cm from incision	Bloody purulent	Skin, subcutaneous fat, and fascial layer separation

Adapted from Davidson N: REEDA: Evaluating postpartum healing. J Nurse-Midwifery 19(2):6-8, 1974.

     e. Ability of mother to understand infant's needs and respond to those needs

     f. Ability of mother to demonstrate or verbalize a positive perception of her infant

     g. Feeding of infant

  4. Consider the following in assessment:

     a. The time after delivery—particularly in relation to mother's physical condition, fatigue level, and pain level—may heavily influence observations.

     b. The habit of looking only for negative characteristics should be avoided.

     c. Cultural variations may influence observations.[10,67,71]

     d. Ongoing assessment is necessary, particularly when possible deviations from normal are noted.

     e. Labeling an interaction as maladaptive must not be done on the basis of a short observation time.

     f. Infant feeding and bathing periods offer some of the most reliable opportunities for observation of parental behavior.[17]

G. Management and teaching

  1. Vital signs

     a. Ensure that appropriate type and interval are ordered for each mother.

     b. Immediately postdelivery:

       • Take temperature once during immediate postpartum period.[66]

       • Several regimens for taking blood pressure and pulse are popular

        — Take blood pressure and pulse every 15 minutes after delivery until stable at predelivery levels—more frequently if indicated,[66]
          or

        — Take blood pressure every 15 minutes for 2 hours, every half hour for 2 hours, and every hour for 3 hours—more frequently if indicated.[69]

     c. Routine care: Make sure that the following occur:

       • Temperature, pulse, and respirations are taken every 4 hours while woman is awake and blood pressure is taken once daily while in hospital or birth center.

       • Mothers discharged prior to 24 hours or mothers delivering at home should take their temperatures every 4 hours while awake for 2 days after delivery.

  2. Diet and fluid intake

     a. Order appropriate diet. Cultural group preferences should be taken into consideration.

     b. Routine care is regular diet without restrictions.

     c. Intake of fluids should be encouraged to prevent constipation, facilitate milk production if breast-feeding, and prevent urinary tract problems.

  3. Activity and rest

     a. Order activity level appropriate for each mother.

    b. Routine care is ambulatory without restrictions.

    c. Instruct mother in appropriate postpartum restoration exercises for abdomen and perineum.[49]

4. Routine laboratory tests

    a. Order hematocrit after 16 hours postpartum.

- Hematocrit determinations within 8 hours of delivery will miss the peak drop in a majority of mothers.
- A drop of less than 10 percent of predelivery value requires no further determination.
- A drop of greater than 10 percent of predelivery values should be repeated at 24 hours postdelivery and then as indicated if the 24-hour value is lower than the 16-hour value.
- Hematocrit values obtained less than 16 hours postpartum due to early discharge should be interpreted cautiously and provisions made for a repeat determination if necessary. Hematocrits on early discharge mothers should be done at 2nd- or 3rd-day postpartum visit.[47]

    b. Initiate evaluation for need for Rh(D) immune globulin (human) if mother is Rh negative.

- Notify mother if she is not a candidate for Rh (D) immune globulin administration.
- If mother is a candidate for Rh (D) immune globulin administration, inform mother, answer questions and administer Rh (D) immune globulin intramuscularly within 72 hours of delivery.
- Document administration of Rh (D) immune globulin or lack of necessity for Rh (D) immune globulin on medical record prior to mother's discharge from hospital or birth center.
- If mother has delivered at home and is a candidate for Rh (D) immune globulin administration, ensure that mother obtains Rh (D) immune globulin within 72 hours of delivery.

The usual dosage of Rh (D) immune globulin is one vial. However, one vial will only suppress the immune response to 15 ml of Rh-positive red blood cells. If a large fetal-maternal hemorrhage is suspected, further laboratory testing should be done to determine the number of vials needed.

---

5. Breast and nipple care: teach mother the importance of the following[37]:

    a. A supportive bra, without plastic liners, worn at all times

    b. Careful hand washing prior to handling of breasts and nipples

    c. Washing breasts with plain water, and no more than once daily[48]

    d. Adequate air drying of nipples after breast-feeding

6. Routine perineal care

    a. Instruct mother in proper perineal hygiene.

- Rinse perineum with warm water, spraying from front to back, after each urination or defecation until lochia diminishes and episiotomy and perineal lacerations have healed.

- Blot gently with tissue from front to back to dry.
- Shower or bathe daily.
- Apply perineal pads from front to back.

b. Apply ice packs to perineum on all mothers (including those with no episiotomy or laceration) immediately postdelivery for 1 hour to minimize edema and pain. To maximize therapeutic effect, ice should be applied for 30-60 minutes then discontinued for 1 hour before reapplication. Longer periods of cold application lead to a phenomenon called *secondary effect*, which reduces the therapeutic effect.[14]

c. Standard management is good perineal hygiene only, unless mother is experiencing pain.

d. Alternative management includes the following:
- Warm sitz baths for all mothers with episiotomy or perineal lacerations, one to four times daily
- Cold sitz baths one to four times daily for mothers experiencing perineal pain[5,16,51]: contraindicated in women with hypertensive disorders or collagen disease

7. Bowel function
   a. Encourage ambulation and adequate fluid intake.
   b. Give Milk of Magnesia, 30 ml orally as needed.
   c. Give ducosate sodium (Colace) 100 mg orally twice daily, for mothers with third- and fourth-degree lacerations.

8. Pain relief
   a. Determine source of pain and institute appropriate nonmedicinal pain relief measures.
   b. Give acetaminophen, 325 mg, one to two tablets orally every 3-4 hours as necessary for pain, or acetaminophen, 325 mg, and codeine 30 mg, one to two tablets orally every 3-4 hours as necessary for pain.

9. Guidelines for care of normal breast-feeding mothers[37]
   a. Infants should be put to breast as soon after birth as possible.
   b. Every mother should be instructed in proper latch-on technique, positioning, and removal, and evaluated before discharge to ensure proper technique is being practiced.
   c. Each mother will receive written information on how the breast functions and instructions for breast-feeding, including information on let-down and the principles of supply and demand.
   d. All babies who do not remain at their mother's bedside will be taken to their mothers on demand or at least every 2½-3 hours around the clock, mother's condition permitting.
   e. No supplementary water or milk will be given unless specifically ordered by a physician or nurse practitioner.
   f. If supplements are ordered, they are to be administered via slow syringe to avoid nipple confusion.
   g. To avoid nipple confusion, pacifiers will not be used unless specifically requested by the mother.

h. Suckling time at each feeding should be at least 7-10 minutes on each side, not including let-down nursing time.

i. Infants should feed from both breasts at all feedings, alternating starting side to stimulate milk supply. Mothers should be instructed that once milk supply is established, infant may be satisfied with only one breast at a feeding.

j. Mothers who must be separated from their babies will be instructed on how to maintain lactation.

k. Follow-up telephone calls within 24-48 hours after delivery or discharge will be made by appropriate personnel.

l. Follow-up appointments for all breast-feeding mothers should be made within 1 week of delivery.

m. Mothers should be given a 24-hour telephone number to call should problems arise and should be encouraged to use it.

n. Breast-feeding mothers should be encouraged to continue taking one prenatal vitamin daily while breast-feeding, to increase oral fluids to 8-12 cups of liquid per day, and to increase calorie intake by at least 500 calories.

o. Instruction sheets for mothers for common breast-feeding problems should be available.

p. Adequate milk intake by infant can be monitored by observing for six to eight wet diapers daily and a content baby who sleeps for 1½-2 hours after feeding.

q. A newborn's refusal to eat during two separate feedings in a row may be a sign of illness and should be reported to the health care provider immediately.

r. The father's support of a mother's decision to breast-feed is a key factor in successful breast-feeding, so his opinion and degree of support should be assessed.

s. Mothers should be instructed to avoid all medications prior to consultation with a health care provider.

10. Guidelines for care of bottle-feeding mothers

a. Lactation suppression instructions will be given to the mother as soon as possible after delivery.[70] These include the following:

- Wear a good snugly fitting bra starting within 6 hours after delivery for 24 hours a day until tenderness or engorgement subsides.
- Do not express any milk.
- Avoid excessive stimulation of breasts and nipples for 1 week (such as from burping baby over the mother's shoulder or allowing water to run over the breasts while showering).
- Apply ice packs to breasts prophylactically (icepack placed over axillary area of breasts for 15-20 minutes at least four times a day for 5 days postpartum) or to already engorged breasts for pain relief.
- Prescribe acetaminophen for pain relief.
- Alternative management: in case of severe engorgement, woman may

mechanically express milk to the point of comfort as necessary, carefully avoiding nipple stimulation.[44]
- Do not limit fluid intake.
b. Lactation suppressants are not given routinely. They may be given when individual situations warrant their use after consultation with a physician. Instruct mother of possibility of rebound lactation at 10-14 days postpartum with the use of lactation suppressants.

Use of hormones has been found to increase the risk of thromboembolic disease in the puerperium.[33,58]

- Chlorotrianisene (TACE): use one of the following recommended dosages:
  — One 12-mg capsule four times a day for 7 days
  — Two 25-mg capsules every 6 hours for 6 doses
  — One 72-mg capsule every 12 hours for 2 days, or
- Deladumone: 4 ml administered intramuscularly at time of delivery, or
- Bromocriptine mescylate (Parlodel): one 2.5-mg tablet twice daily for 14 days, with meals
  — Rebound lactation may be treated with an extra week of medication. Side effects such as nausea and vomiting, headache, dizziness, and hypertension have been reported in up to 40 percent of medicated mothers.
  — Postpartum myocardial infarction, seizures, and cerebrovascular accidents are also under investigation as being associated with bromocriptine use.[31,34]
c. Provide bottle-feeding instructions for mother:
  - Feed baby every 3-4 hours for 15-30 minutes.
  - Feed formula at room temperature. Formula should be refrigerated after preparation then brought to room temperature prior to feeding.
  - Newborn formula requirements range from 11-22 ounces of formula per 24-hour period depending on size of the infant.
  - Tilt bottle so nipple is always filled with formula.
  - Burp baby several times during feeding.
  - Never prop the bottle or put the baby to bed with a bottle, to avoid bottle-mouth syndrome.
11. Parent-infant interaction[13,35]
  a. Opportunities for enhancing positive, pleasant parent-infant interactions, both for father and mother, should be actively sought and used to full advantage.
    - Keep mother's physical comfort level at as optimum a level as possible.
    - Maximize parent-infant contact time and opportunities for caregiving activities.

- Provide for nursing assistance during feeding periods.
- Provide instruction, anticipatory guidance, and serve as role model whenever necessary. Avoid using the professional role in a way that may be demeaning to or discouraging of parental efforts.
- Keep parents updated on infant condition.
- Use infant exams to acquaint parents with their infant and teach infant characteristics and behavior. (Some settings use the Brazelton Neonatal Behavioral Assessment scale for this purpose[4,9])

b. Assist parents to put perceived negative infant responses or negative unpleasant interactions into proper perspective.
c. Use all possible opportunities to encourage and praise parental efforts, build confidence, and strengthen parental problem-solving abilities.

II. Management of common postpartum problems

A. Afterpains
  1. History and physical exam
    a. Determine whether afterpains are continuous or only occur during nursing.
    b. Palpate uterus to rule out abnormality or unusual tenderness.
  2. Management and teaching[57]
    a. Instruct mother to empty bladder frequently, especially prior to breast-feeding, to allow uterus to contract efficiently.
    b. Instruct mother to gently massage her uterus or lie in a prone position with a small pillow under abdomen.
    c. Instruct mother to place ice bag firmly against uterus for 10 minutes.
    d. Provide pain medication, preferably aspirin or acetaminophen, as necessary if above measures are inadequate. (There is conflicting information in the literature regarding the effectiveness of codeine for afterpains.) Medication 30 minutes prior to breast-feeding is helpful if pain occurs while nursing.
    e. Consult physician for severe uterine cramping unrelieved by above measures or for unusual uterine tenderness.
    f. Follow-up: relief due to comfort measures and a gradually diminishing intensity of pain should be observed and documented before the mother is released from health care supervision.

B. Breast engorgement
  1. Clinical features
    a. Enlargement of breasts
    b. Shiny, reddened, taut, warm skin
    c. Tenderness, pain, and throbbing sensations
    d. Breasts are firm, lumpy, or hard to the touch
  2. Management and teaching
    a. Management for bottle-feeding mothers (see Section I, G, 10)
    b. Management for breast-feeding mothers

- Explain the reason and expected duration of engorgement to mother.
- Observe mother breastfeeding to be sure improper breastfeeding technique is not contributing to the problem.
- Advise mother to feed frequently, at least every 2½ hours for 15-20 minutes per side.
- Advise mother to apply moist heat to breasts prior to feeding, using hot packs or shower, and to lightly stroke skin from outer edges of breasts towards areola with a fine-toothed baby comb to enhance let-down reflex while showering (Naylor A: Empirical management used by midwives in Brazil. Personal communication. 1986.).
- Teach mother to manually express milk prior to feeding to soften areolar area.
- Encourage mother to massage breasts from outer edges to areola during feeding. With severe pain, mother may be unable to do this herself and may need assistance until engorgement subsides. Lotion can be used to reduce skin friction while massaging.
- Encourage mother to use a good supportive bra.
- Mother should apply ice packs to breasts between feedings.
- Medicate mother 30 minutes prior to feeding to enhance relaxation.
- Observe carefully for development of sore nipples.
- Mechanical breast pump can be used after baby nurses if baby is small or sleepy and not emptying breasts effectively.
- Give mother written instructions for management of engorgement.
- Reexamine mother 6-12 hours after relief measures have been instituted to ensure effectiveness of comfort measures and observe for diminishing severity of engorgement.

C. Low hematocrit
  1. History
    a. Determine presence or absence of dizziness and extent.
    b. Elicit feeling of fatigue and presence of headaches.
    c. Determine amount of postpartum bleeding.
  2. Physical exam
    a. Evaluate for sources of ongoing blood loss.
    b. Evaluate for orthostatic changes in pulse and blood pressure.
  3. Laboratory studies: repeat hematocrit as necessary to detect peak drop in hematocrit value
  4. Management and teaching
    a. Encourage adequate fluid intake and rest.
    b. Prescribe ferrous sulfate, 300 mg orally with meals, three times a day until 6 week examination.
    c. Counsel mother on constipating effects of iron and ways to avoid them, on use of iron-rich foods, and on susceptibility to infection while anemic.
    d. Consult with physician for the following:

- Significant changes in hematocrit
- Excessively low hematocrit
- Continued presence of orthostatic changes and dizziness
- Hematocrit that continues to drop
- Possible need for blood transfusion for hematocrit lower than 29 percent at altitude of 5000 feet or 25 percent at sea level; if the mother is able to function, a decision to transfuse will often not be made, unless the hematocrit is even lower, due to risk of infectious disease transmission via blood products

  e. Check hematocrit at 6 week postpartum examination.

D. Hemorrhoids
  1. Nonpainful hemorrhoids
     a. Explain the condition to the mother along with the need for good health habits to avoid flare-ups.
     b. Teach measures to avoid constipation: adequate fluid intake, dietary fiber, adequate rest and exercise, establishment of regular bowel habits.
     c. Suggest placing both feet on a small stool while defecating to maintain a more physiological position for bowel evacuation.
     d. Teach Kegel exercises to improve blood flow to the area.
  2. Painful hemorrhoids[39]
     a. Provide same teaching as for the mother with nonpainful hemorrhoids.
     b. Apply ice pack to hemorrhoids for 30-60 minutes then discontinue for 1 hour. Reapply as necessary.
     c. Use warm sitz baths if no relief from ice.
     d. Apply local anesthetic ointments or sprays (Epifoam, Americaine).
     e. Medicate for pain as necessary.
     f. Order hemorrhoidal creams or suppositories, especially those containing hydrocortisone.
     g. Reinsert external hemorrhoids if possible and maintain position by Kegel exercises.
     h. A stool softener or a bulk-forming laxative may be ordered to avoid constipation, e.g., ducosate sodium, 100 mg orally twice daily, or psyllium hydrophilic mucilloid 1 rounded teaspoonful in 8 ounces of liquid orally one to three times daily.
     i. Mother should lie down with hips elevated.
  3. Consult for extensive or thrombosed hemorrhoids or for severe pain that is unrelieved by above measures; anal dilation (Lord's procedure), incision of thrombosed hemorrhoids, or hemorrhoidectomy may be necessary.
  4. Reinforce teaching at postpartum visits to reduce the incidence of further problems.

E. Nipple soreness
  1. Prevention
     a. Provide assistance to mother at initial feedings to teach proper breast-feeding technique.

    b. Teach and encourage proper nipple care and hygiene.

    c. Medical or nursing personnel should examine nipples daily while mother is in hospital or birth center and at each home or clinic visit to detect early problems.

    d. Reevaluate breast-feeding technique prior to release of mother from health care supervision.

2. History

    a. Determine amount of pain and when it occurs.

    b. Inquire about proper latch-on and breaking of suction before removing baby from breast and use of alternate breasts at subsequent feedings.

    c. Determine frequency and duration of nursing.

    d. Note comfort measures already used.

    e. Elicit technique for care of nipples: use of soap, too frequent washing.

3. Physical exam

    a. Examine nipples for redness, blisters, cracks or fissures, bleeding.

    b. Assess breasts for presence and extent of engorgement.

    c. Observe feeding to detect improper technique, vigorous nurser.

4. Management and teaching

    a. Reassure mother the condition is short-lived and correctable.

    b. Observe nursing technique to determine cause of problem.

    c. Medicate mother prior to nursing if necessary and teach relaxation techniques.

    d. Review proper latch-on of baby or correct improper latch-on to ensure areola is well into baby's mouth.

    e. Stimulate let-down reflex prior to putting the baby to breast.

    f. Nurse on least painful side first.

    g. Teach mother to vary baby's position to change pressure from most painful areas.

    h. Teach mother how to break suction before taking baby away from the breast.

    i. Mother should breast-feed about every 2 hours for shorter time periods, but always at least 5-10 minutes after let-down.

    j. Air-dry nipples well after nursing, expose to air and/or sunlight as much as possible.

    k. Apply breast milk, hydrous lanolin, or other nipple cream to areolar area after air-drying to promote healing. Instruct mother to avoid putting ointment on tip of nipple which would clog ducts.

    l. Rinse nipples no more than once daily with plain water; use no soap on nipples or areolae.

    m. For severe pain, apply cloth-wrapped ice cubes to nipples for 5-10 minutes prior to nursing to numb area.

    n. If pain is severe, mother may discontinue nursing for 24-48 hours on affected side if breasts are manually or mechanically emptied every 2 hours.

    o. Avoid use of nipple shields to eliminate nipple confusion and to avoid prolonging the pain of sore nipples.

    p. Provide follow-up management.
- Assistance with nursing should be immediately available during period of most severe pain.
- Do not release mother from health care supervision, either in person or by telephone, until proper nursing technique is consistently used, relief due to comfort measures is noted, and amount of nipple pain has diminished.
- Provide telephone follow-up within 24-48 hours of discharge from hospital or birth center.
- Schedule visit for mother and infant 5-7 days after discharge.

F. Perineal edema and pain
1. History: determine onset, duration, location, and intensity of pain
2. Physical exam
    a. Carefully examine perineum for presence and degree of redness, edema, ecchymosis, discharge, and approximation of any wound edges (see Section I, D, 7). Palpate for induration or oozing of purulent material from wound edges.
    b. Document findings precisely for comparison of improvement over time.
    c. Perform gentle vaginal or rectal exam if any indication that pain is due to hematoma formation, i.e., bulging tissue, increasing pain, systemic signs of continuing blood loss.
3. Management and teaching
    a. Apply ice pack to perineum first hour after delivery for prevention.
    b. Teach perineal hygiene to ensure area is kept clean and dry (see I, G, 6).
    c. Apply ice pack to perineum 30-60 minutes, then discontinue for 1 hour and repeat as necessary for pain.[14]
    d. Use warm sitz bath one to four times daily for 15 minutes. An alternate management is the use of cold sitz bath one to four times daily for 10-15 minutes[5,16,51]
    e. Teach gentle tightening of perineal muscles (Kegel exercise) to draw wound edges together, mobilize edema, and restore circulation to area.[49] Vigorous perineal muscle exercises should be avoided for first few days or when a third- or fourth-degree laceration is present.
    f. Apply magnesium sulfate soaks to episiotomy, lacerations, or edematous areas continuously until swelling decreases.[45]
    g. Provide witch hazel soaks, anesthetic ointments, or anesthetic sprays as necessary.
    h. Teach perineal splinting to reduce strain on tissues during defecation.[52]
    i. Medicate with aspirin or acetaminophen, 325 mg, one to two tablets orally every 3-4 hours as necessary, with or without codeine, 30 mg
    j. Encourage measures to avoid constipation (see Section II, D).
    k. Consult physician for the following[20,62]:
- Extensive vulvar or perineal edema

- Discharge other than serous oozing
- *Any* degree of induration
- Severe pain unrelieved by comfort measures
- Dehiscence of wound edges
- Evidence of hematoma formation
- Fever not explained by other physical findings

l. Provide follow-up management
- Release mother from health care supervision when the following occur:
  — Relief from comfort measures is noted.
  — Intensity of pain diminishes.
  — Improvement in physical findings is observed.
- Do the following at the 6 week examination:
  — Examine healed episiotomy or laceration for good anatomical results.
  — Check for integrity of perineal muscles and rectal sphincter.
  — Emphasize need for daily Kegel exercises to maintain good condition of perineal muscles.

G. Postpartum "blues"
1. Prevention
   a. Encourage mother to make plans for how she will manage the demands on her time postpartum.
   b. Provide concrete suggestions for pregnant women and mothers postpartum to help in the adjustment to motherhood.[25]
   - Get as much help from the baby's father, family, and friends as possible.
   - Get as much rest as possible. Nap while the baby naps.
   - Maintain outside interests but cut down on responsibilities and time commitments.
   - Arrange for babysitters and locate a doctor for the baby early.
   - Make friends with other people with children.
   - Relax housekeeping standards and avoid unimportant tasks.
   c. Include a description of the symptoms of postpartum blues in postpartum teaching and discharge instructions.
   d. Assess for factors predisposing mother to postpartum depression (other than baby blues).[7,24]
   - Previous history of depression or postpartum depression/psychosis
   - Depression during pregnancy
   - History of postpartum depression in a close family member
   - Expression of often feeling unloved by father of child
   - Unplanned and/or unwanted pregnancy
   - Single or separated
   - Admission of marital problems
   e. Pregnant women with a personal or family history of depression should receive prenatal counseling about the signs and symptoms of depression.

    f. Provide as much emotional support throughout pregnancy, delivery, and postpartum as possible to women identified as high risk for depression.

    g. Postpartum women with a previous history of depression or previous or family history of postpartum depression/psychosis should be seen biweekly between the 2nd and 6th postpartum week for evaluation of depression.[24]

2. Assessment

    a. Be aware that many normal physiological changes of the puerperium are similar to symptoms of depression (lack of sexual interest, appetite change, fatigue).

    b. Mother may or may not recognize the presence of symptoms herself.

    c. Telephone calls from mothers about vague concerns or unusual or inappropriate questions (such as calls about vitamins at 2 o'clock in the morning) should be viewed as an indication to inquire about postpartum blues and to assess mother's coping abilities.

    d. Assess type, severity, and duration of symptoms.
- Fatigue
- Crying
- Anxiety
- Irritability/mood changes
- Poor concentration, forgetfulness
- Sleeping difficulties
- Appetite change

    e. Identify any specific problems that mother feels are contributing to her distress.

3. Differential diagnosis

    a. Postpartum blues, baby blues: transitory minor affective disorder occurring during the first few postpartum days

    b. Chronic depressive syndrome or moderate depression disorder

    c. Postpartum reaction syndrome (including schizophrenia, psychoneurosis, and depression)

4. Management

    a. Identify presence of postpartum blues symptoms to mother.

    b. Give mother adequate time, opportunity, and encouragement to express her feelings.

    c. Reassure mother that although condition is distressing, it is normal, short-lived, and will disappear spontaneously.

    d. Encourage mother to accept or request help with housework and child care from family and friends.

    e. Encourage mother to use relaxation techniques learned in childbirth classes to relieve distress or teach mother relaxation techniques.[27]

    f. Help mother to develop solutions or give mother specific suggestions for solving any specific problems she has identified.

    g. Encourage mother to call again if she needs to talk or if symptoms persist.

5. Follow-up management
   a. Telephone mother in 24-48 hours to check for improvement.
   b. Refer to a mental health professional for any of the following:
- Prenatally for women with a previous history of depression or family history of postpartum depression
- Rejection of infant
- Physical aggression against the infant or threat of aggression
- Depressive symptoms from four of the following categories that present daily for 2 or more weeks[24]:
    — Appetite or weight change
    — Insomnia or hypersomnia
    — Psychomotor agitation or retardation
    — Loss of interest or pleasure in usual activities
    — Loss of energy
    — Feelings of worthlessness or guilt
    — Difficulty concentrating or making decisions
    — Thoughts of death or suicide
   c. Assess for persistence of symptoms at 6 week postpartum examination.
H. Sleeping
  1. Encourage mother to nap frequently during the day to compensate for sleep lost at night. Resting quietly is also helpful even if sleep is not possible.
  2. Hospital or birth center routines and visiting hours should be organized to maximize opportunities for rest. Personnel should be encouraged to postpone all but the most critical treatments or medications if a mother is asleep. Encourage mother to limit visitors at home and disconnect phone while napping, to minimize sleep interruption.
  3. Medicate mother for pain, which may be a contributing factor.
  4. Teach progressive relaxation techniques.
  5. Sedatives may be ordered for difficulty sleeping while in the hospital if all other methods have failed. Sedatives should not be given to breast-feeding mothers due to transmission in breast milk. Sedative use in bottle-feeding mothers may interfere with normal interaction between mother and infant.
I. Voiding
  1. Prevention
   a. Palpate for distended bladder often in early postpartum period, particularly in mothers with long labors, traumatic deliveries, oxytocin augmentation, perineal edema, extensive episiotomy or lacerations, or regional anesthesia.[41,68]
   b. Encourage early and frequent voiding after delivery.
   c. Encourage adequate fluid intake.
   d. Teach signs and symptoms of urinary tract infection.
  2. History
   a. Inability to void, amounts voided, frequency of voiding
   b. Amount of bleeding

    c. Amount of pain experienced and location

3. Physical exam: palpate uterus and bladder to determine extent of problem and establish baseline physical findings

4. Management and teaching

    a. Medicate mother prior to attempting voiding if mother is experiencing pain or may be unaware that mild pain may be contributing to the problem.

    b. Instruct mother to attempt voiding every 2 hours while awake whether an urge to void is present or not.

    c. Have mother try to void in shower, in warm sitz bath, or while pouring warm water over perineum.

    d. Measure and record output to ensure satisfactory emptying—at least 100 ml.

    e. Recheck position of uterus and bladder immediately after voiding attempt.

    f. Catheterize promptly if bladder is distended and all attempts to help mother void have failed.[29]

    g. If mother continues to void in amounts less than 100 ml after the above methods have been tried, catheterize for residual volume.
- An indwelling catheter should be placed for 24 hours if the amount of residual urine is greater than 150 ml.
- Obtain urine culture prior to discontinuing catheter.
- Bladder training prior to discontinuing catheter (clamp for 2 hours and drain; repeat sequence one time to simulate normal function) is ordered by many physicians but is felt to be ineffective by most urologists.

    h. Consult with physician if the following occurs:
- Mother is unable to void after an indwelling catheter has been used.
- A fever develops.
- A positive urine culture is taken.
- An indwelling catheter is in place greater than 24 hours, for possible prophylactic antibiotic therapy.[28,29]

    i. Follow-up management
- Release from health care supervision when the following occur: ·
  — Voiding is in amounts greater than 100 ml without difficulty.
  — Vaginal bleeding is normal.
  — Uterus is appropriately positioned relative to postpartum day.
- Six week postpartum management of mothers who had an indwelling catheter more than 24 hours is as follows:
  — Question carefully about urinary tract symptoms.
  — Consider urinalysis and/or urine culture.

III. Management of common postpartum complications

A. **Infectious mastitis**

    1. Prevention[21]

    a. Avoid engorgement and stasis of milk caused by missed feedings or abrupt weaning.

    b. Teach mother proper breast-feeding techniques to minimize problems with sore, cracked nipples or engorgement.

    c. Explain let-down reflex to mother and its importance to successful breast-feeding.

    d. Teach signs and symptoms of mastitis and stress importance of early reporting of any symptoms.

2. History

    a. Malaise, flu-like feeling, muscle pain

    b. Fever and/or chills

    c. Diaphoresis

    d. Headache

    e. Problems with breast-feeding

    f. Sore or cracked nipples

    g. Change in feeding pattern

    h. Painful breasts

3. Physical exam

    a. Take temperature and pulse.

    b. Examine breasts for the following:
   - Tenderness, swelling, redness
   - Warmth, either generalized or localized

    c. Examine nipples for the following:
   - Cracks or fissures
   - Redness
   - Type of discharge
   - Bleeding

4. Laboratory studies

    a. Need for laboratory studies such as culture and antibody sensitivity studies in the treatment of mastitis is controversial, and management is usually based on history and physical findings only.

    b. The use of leukocyte and bacterial counts per milliliter of breast milk has been suggested as a means of differential diagnosis.[64,65]

    c. Obtain milk specimen, if determined necessary, by cleansing nipple, allowing to dry, hand expressing several milliliters of milk, and then collecting one of the following squirts of milk.

5. Differential diagnosis

    a. Milk stasis: short duration, mild symptoms usually with a good outcome regardless of treatment, and mother is usually afebrile.

    b. Noninfectious inflammation of the breast: more severe inflammatory symptoms persisting for several days.

    c. Infectious mastitis: most persistent and least likely to resolve without therapy, mother is usually febrile, visibly ill, and in pain.

6. Management of milk stasis, noninfectious inflammation of the breast, and infectious mastitis

a. Tell the mother to do the following:
  • Get as much bed rest as possible.
  • Increase fluid intake to 2-3 quarts daily.
  • Feed baby as frequently as possible, at least every 2-2 ½ hours for 15-20 minutes per side. If mother wants to discontinue nursing, encourage her to delay doing so, or at least to pump her breasts to avoid abscess formation until infection is controlled.
  • Apply warm compresses to breast.
  • Massage breast from periphery toward nipple during feedings.
  • Take aspirin, 650 mg or acetaminophen, 650 mg, orally, if necessary for pain, every 4 hours.
  • Take temperature every 4 hours.
b. Assess possible contributing factors to development of mastitis and correct poor nursing technique:
  • Cracked nipples
  • Poor hygiene
  • Engorgement
  • Change in mother's routine or infant feeding patterns leading to poor or irregular emptying of breast
  • Supplemental feeding
  • Abrupt weaning
c. Consult physician regarding the need for antibiotic therapy. Progression of milk stasis and noninfectious inflammation of the breast to infectious mastitis may sometimes be prevented by aggressive use of the treatment measures listed above without antibiotics, but must be closely monitored. Mothers with full-blown signs and symptoms of mastitis should be immediately treated with penicillinase-resistant penicillin.
d. Consult physician for failure to respond to treatment or for suspected abscess formation.
e. Provide follow-up management.
  • Contact mother within 24 hours of beginning of treatment to determine effectiveness.
  • Assess resolution of breast-feeding problems contributing to mastitis.
7. Teaching
a. Explain condition, treatment, preventive measures, and lack of negative effects on infant.
b. Give mother written instructions for care of mastitis.
c. Tell mother to contact care provider if no improvement in 6-8 hours or immediately if fever worsens.
d. Encourage slow, gradual weaning, when weaning is desired, to avoid problems with mastitis.
B. **Maternal hematoma in the postpartum period**
1. Prevention techniques:
a. Control of pregnancy-induced hypertension
b. Careful attention to delivery technique

    c. Careful use of oxytocics to avoid precipitous delivery

    d. Ligation of specific bleeding points during episiotomy/laceration repair

    e. Good tissue approximation and placement of first suture above apex of vaginal mucosa of episiotomy

    f. Careful and frequent inspection of vaginal area, episiotomy, and lacerations after delivery and in the first 4 hours postpartum to ensure good hemostasis

2. History

    a. Presence of perineal, vaginal, or rectal pressure

    b. Amount, character, and intensity of pain

    c. Difficulty voiding or inability to void

    d. Presence of uterine, abdominal, or flank pain.

3. Physical exam

    a. Swelling of vulva, ecchymosis, extent

    b. Amount of bleeding

    c. Abdominal distension

    d. Signs and symptoms of shock

    e. Hematocrit recheck for signs of ongoing blood loss

    f. Low grade fever and tachycardia

    g. Rectal and/or vaginal exam if there is severe pain to rule out possibility of concealed hematoma

4. Management of small vulvar hematomas and teaching

    a. Observe closely for enlargement of hematoma.

    b. Apply ice packs and pressure.

    c. Administer analgesics. Inspect perineum prior to administration of pain medication when pain is persistent or severe to rule out enlarging hematoma.

    d. Monitor blood pressure and pulse closely.

    e. Catheterize if unable to void.

    f. Explain nature and cause of problem to patient and describe treatment.

    g. Provide consultation and referral.[30]

      • Consult with physician for vaginal hematomas.

      • Refer to physician for the following:

        — Persistent bleeding

        — Suspected subperitoneal hematoma

        — Large vulvar or vaginal hematomas

        — Signs and symptoms of impending shock

        — Significant fall in hematocrit

    h. Provide follow-up: Monitor hematocrit to document control of bleeding.

C. **Mild pregnancy-induced hypertension**

1. Postpartum Management

    a. Onset in postpartum period: consult with physician

    b. Onset in labor

      • Continue maintenance doses of magnesium sulfate for 24 hours postpartum.

- Check blood pressure and respirations every 4 hours.
- Assess deep tendon reflexes, presence or absence of clonus, and mother's subjective symptoms every 12 hours, more frequently if indicated by mother's condition or symptoms.
- After physician consultation, discontinue magnesium sulfate after 24 hours if blood pressure and deep tendon reflexes are within normal limits.
- Monitor urinary output while on magnesium sulfate therapy.
- Consult physician for no improvement or worsening of vital signs, deep tendon reflexes, or subjective symptoms.

2. Teaching
   a. Ensure mother's understanding of condition, treatment, signs and symptoms, and need for rest.
   b. Stress importance of periodic blood pressure evaluations and need to alert medical personnel of diagnosis during subsequent pregnancies.

3. Follow-up
   a. Evaluate blood pressure at 2 weeks postpartum if elevated at time of discharge. Consult if elevated.
   b. Evaluate blood pressure at 6 week postpartum examination.
   c. Refer mothers with elevated blood pressure readings at 6 weeks for evaluation of possible chronic hypertension.

D. **Postpartum infection**
   1. Prevention techniques[38]
      a. Promoting adequate nutrition, prenatal care, and hygiene in all pregnant women
      b. Rigid adherence to good hand-washing and aseptic technique by all health care personnel
      c. Facilitation of normal processes of labor to minimize need for operative intervention
      d. Careful physical examination and monitoring of vital signs for 2-3 days postpartum either by health care personnel or by mothers taught to take their temperature, assess their physical condition, and watch for symptoms or complications
   2. Preliminary management
      a. In first 24 hours, if temperature is up to 100.4° F, do the following:
         - Force fluids, 1000 ml or more in 2-3 hours.
         - Retake temperature every 4 hours around the clock.
      b. If temperature is greater than 100.4° F, or if mother was febrile in labor, do the following:
         - Check for sources of fever as described for after 24 hours, (see below).
         - Force fluids.
         - Consult physician.
      c. After 24 hours for elevated temperatures or persistent low-grade fever,[1,18,22] do the following:

- Review medical record for predisposing factors, antepartum or intrapartum problems, postpartum course to date, and medications.
- Question mother about possible signs and symptoms including the following:
  — General: headache, malaise, general achiness, flu-like symptoms, stiff neck
  — Dental—abscessed tooth, toothache.
  — Gastrointestinal: nausea, vomiting, diarrhea, anorexia
  — Upper respiratory: cough, sore throat, runny nose, sneezing, earache
  — Breast: pain, tenderness, hardening, heat, discoloration
  — Chest: chest pain, shortness of breath
  — Uterus: amount, character, color, and odor of lochia, presence and intensity of afterbirth pains; tenderness of uterus, presence of clots
  — Urinary tract: dysuria, frequency, urgency, difficulty voiding, back or suprapubic pain, unusual odor or color of urine, amount of urine
  — Perineum, vulva, and vagina: pain, swelling
  — Lower extremities: pain, redness, tenderness, warmth or coolness of skin
  — Skin: rashes, itching
- Determine the following:
  — Fluid intake since delivery, especially for fever in the first 24 hours
  — For breast-feeding mothers: problems with nursing, difficulty with let-down, presence of engorgement, unusual nursing patterns, condition of nipples
  — Current medications and when each was started; reactions to any drugs taken previously
  — Any recent illness in mother, family members, or friends
- Review vital signs.
- Perform a thorough physical examination, including the following:
  — HEENT (head, eyes, ears, nose, throat): caries or abscessed teeth, condition of tonsils and throat; pain from pressure over sinus areas; condition of tympanic membranes; lymphadenopathy; nuchal rigidity or pain on flexion of neck; condition of eyegrounds
  — Lungs: presence of rales or rhonchi
  — Breasts: consistency, masses, tenderness, discoloration, warmth; discharge from nipple, nipple condition
  — Abdomen and back: softness or rigidity; tenderness (direct or rebound); character of bowel sounds; masses, inguinal nodes; presence or absence of distension; location, consistency, and tenderness of uterus (compare with previous findings); for mothers who have had a cesarean section or tubal ligation: condition of incision, color, induration, discharge from wound, tenderness

— Perineum: swelling, redness, edema, ecchymosis, induration, character and odor of discharge or exudate; approximation of stitches; color, odor, and amount of lochia
— Lower extremities and skin: tenderness; discoloration, warmth, or coolness of skin; swelling; presence and condition of varicosities; Homan's sign; measure girth of calves and thighs if indicated

3. Consultation and referral
    a. Consult with physician regarding history and physical findings.
    b. Depending on local preference, physician will perform pelvic and rectal exam, or direct other health care provider to do so, to assess the following:
       • Presence or absence of foreign body in vagina
       • Condition of internal vaginal sutures
       • Character of drainage from cervical os
       • Condition of cervix and patency of cervical os
       • Size, consistency, and tenderness of uterus
       • Presence or absence of adnexal or other masses or tenderness
       • Integrity of rectovaginal septum and episiotomy/laceration repair
    c. Order and/or perform any lab tests recommended by physician, including the following:
       • Catheterized urine specimen for urinalysis, culture, and sensitivity
       • Endometrial cultures—aerobic and anaerobic and chlamydial—preferably done with a double-lumen protected swab to protect against cervical contamination.[18,19]
       • Complete blood count with differential
       • Other cultures as indicated, such as throat and incisional drainage
       • Blood cultures
    d. Inform pediatrician of temperature elevation.

4. Management after diagnosis
    a. Implement appropriate portions of management plan determined by physician.[18,36]
    b. Explain diagnosis, laboratory test findings, and treatment plan to mother and allow for questions and expression of feelings.
    c. If antibiotic therapy is necessary, inform mother of the need to complete full course of treatment.
    d. Ensure availability of appropriate comfort measures: analgesics and antipyretics; showering and fresh linen for excessive diaphoresis; antihistamines, decongestants, cough medicine for upper respiratory infections, etc.
    e. Monitor vital signs and mother's condition to assure resolution of the problem.
    f. Make sure mother knows the signs and symptoms to watch for should the problem recur.
    g. Arrange for follow-up outpatient examinations or laboratory examinations as indicated.

E. **Postpartum thrombophlebitis: superficial, deep vein, and/or pelvic**[18,56]
   1. Prevention techniques
      a. Maintain good hydration intrapartum and postpartum.
      b. Avoid pressure on legs from stirrups during delivery.
      c. Provide support hose for mothers with varicosities.
      d. Minimize blood loss during delivery and postpartum.
      e. Encourage ambulation in labor and early ambulation postpartum.
      f. Avoid lactation suppressants containing estrogen.
      g. Do not allow oral contraceptives until 10-14 days postpartum.
      h. Maintain good obstetrical and hygiene practices to avoid endometritis.
      i. Facilitate normal parturition to reduce need for obstetrical intervention.
   2. History
      a. Chills, fever
      b. Leg pain
      c. Abdominal pain
      d. General malaise
      e. Chest pain, shortness of breath
   3. Physical exam
      a. Slight to high fever, tachycardia, chills
      b. Abdominal pain, costovertebral angle (CVA) tenderness, abdominal mass, tenderness on pelvic or rectal exam (with pelvic thrombophlebitis)
      c. Local warmth or coolness, redness, tenderness
      d. Edema of leg, ankle, and thigh, distended superficial veins
      e. Calf and thigh girth measurements
      f. Presence or absence of Homan's sign (not always present even with thrombophlebitis)
      g. Sharp chest pain, shortness of breath, tachypnea, dyspnea, respiratory rales, hemoptysis, tachycardia with pulmonary embolus
   4. Referral: immediately if signs of thrombophlebitis occur
   5. Teaching
      a. Teach signs and symptoms to mother, especially those at higher risk of thrombophlebitis, and encourage them to seek medical advice if any symptoms occur.
      b. Venous valves in area of thrombosis are destroyed; mother may need elastic support hose and to avoid positions of stasis to avoid future problems.
   6. Follow-up management
      a. Question mother at 6 week check-up regarding resolution of symptoms and examine for any signs of thrombophlebitis.
      b. Review preventive measures with mother and stress importance of their continued use.
      c. Alert mother to report condition to health care provider in subsequent pregnancies.

F. **Subinvolution**
   1. History since delivery
      a. Uterine tenderness
      b. Prolonged or excessive lochia, prolonged leukorrhea
      c. Delayed bleeding
      d. Fever
      e. Presence of cramps
   2. Physical exam
      a. Perform speculum exam to observe amount and character of lochia.
      b. Perform bimanual examination for position, size, and consistency of uterus, and presence or absence of tenderness.
      c. Take temperature and pulse.
   3. Laboratory studies: hematocrit
   4. Differential diagnosis[50]
      a. Subinvolution
      b. Retained placental fragments
      c. Endometritis
      d. Myomas
   5. Management and teaching
      a. Consult with physician.
         • Order antibiotics if fever is present for suspected endometritis.
         • Order methergine or ergotrate, 0.2 mg orally every 4 hours for 24-48 hours, in presence of large, boggy, nontender uterus, no fever, no foul-smelling uterine discharge, and no bleeding.
      b. Recheck uterine size in 2 weeks. Consult with physician if no improvement.
      c. Explain condition and treatment to mother and stress importance of reexamination.
G. **Urinary tract infection**
   1. Prevention techniques
      a. Screen for and treat antepartum asymptomatic bacteriuria and acute urinary tract infection.
      b. Encourage mother to void frequently in labor and postpartum period to avoid need for catheterization.
      c. Encourage adequate fluid intake.
      d. Observe carefully for bladder distension and inadequate voiding.
      e. Teach proper perineal hygiene.
      f. Avoid routine catheterization at delivery.
   2. History
      a. Dysuria, frequency, urgency, blood in urine
      b. Fever, appetite loss
      c. High fever, chills, nausea and vomiting, abdominal or back pain—with upper urinary tract infection
   3. Physical exam
      a. Take temperature, and pulse.

b. Palpate abdomen and uterus.

c. Perform pelvic exam to rule out uterine pathology.

d. Check for CVA tenderness.

4. Management

a. Obtain clean-voided urine specimen for urinalysis and culture prior to antibiotic therapy.

b. Catheterize for specimen if mother's ability to obtain a clean-voided specimen is impaired.

c. Repeat urine culture if bacterial count is between 10,000 and 100,000.

d. Obtain specific gravity to differentiate between upper and lower urinary tract infection.

e. Consult with physician regarding need for urinary analgesics or antibiotic therapy for cystitis. Timing of antibiotic therapy relative to culture report will depend on severity of patient symptoms.

f. Refer to physician for treatment of symptoms of upper urinary tract infection.

5. Teaching

a. Explain condition and treatment to mother.

b. Encourage increased fluid intake.

c. Encourage frequent voiding.

d. Teach mother to watch for symptoms in future and seek medical help if they occur.

e. Encourage completion of entire course of antibiotics.

6. Follow-up management

a. Observe for response to antibiotics in 24-48 hours.

b. Reculture at 6 week postpartum visit.

c. Review preventive measures with mother.

IV. Discharge of mother from hospital or birth center

A. Assessment

1. Assess mother's knowledge of the following:

a. Self-assessment of physical condition

- Breasts
- Diastasis recti
- Uterine size and position
- Episiotomy or laceration healing
- Legs

b. Self-care

- Need for rest
- Hygiene
- Nutritional needs
- Breast care
- Manual expression of milk for breast-feeding mothers
- Perineal care
- Abdominal and perineal tightening exercises

     c. Infant care
- Feeding technique: breast or bottle, burping.
- Formula preparation and storage
- Diapering and dressing
- Care of cord and circumcision, if applicable
- Bathing
- Taking infant's temperature
- Signs of illness
- Plans for well-baby care

     d. Normal postpartum changes in breasts, perineum, and lochia

     e. Postpartum danger signs and when to call for help
- Fever, chills
- Difficulty voiding
- Abdominal pain
- Difficulties with breast-feeding, including engorgement, sore nipples, or mastitis symptoms
- Excessive bleeding or foul-smelling lochia
- Problems with episiotomy: pain, discharge
- Leg pain
- Persistent headaches
- Depression, inability to care for self or baby

  2. Reassess psychosocial status, support systems, and parent-infant interaction.

  3. Examine breasts, lungs, abdomen, uterine fundus, perineum, lochia, extremities, and review vital signs with all findings within normal limits.

B. Laboratory exam and follow-up

  1. Review hematocrit, rubella titer, Venereal Disease Research Laboratory test (VDRL), Purified Protein Derivative tuberculin antigen test (PPD) (where routine), blood type, and Rh results to ensure that any indicated follow-up or referral has been instituted. Note any unusual medical or obstetric conditions and arrange for appropriate treatment and follow-up, such as postponed chest x-ray, *Trichomonas* vaginal infection untreated in pregnancy, or need for postpartum intravenous pyelogram (IVP).

  2. Arrange for rubella vaccination of nonimmune mothers. Stress importance of avoiding pregnancy for 3 months after vaccination, and document mother's understanding on medical record. (Acute arthritis may develop in 3.7-18.2 percentage of women receiving rubella vaccine in the postpartum period.[63])

  3. Make sure that appropriate newborn procedures and laboratory studies have been done (vitamin K, neonatal opthalmic prophylaxis, phenylketonuria (PKU), hypothyroidism, and galactosemia testing) and that infant is ready for discharge.

C. Teaching

  1. Instruct mother, father, and other family members or friends present in any areas not adequately covered previously.

  2. Discuss the integration of a new baby into the family with other children.

3. Instruct regarding resumption of sexual activity.
   a. No intercourse until bright red bleeding stops, episiotomy or laceration repair is well-healed (about 3 weeks), and both partners feel they are emotionally ready to resume intercourse. (Father will often be the more reluctant partner for fear of causing pain to the mother.)
   b. Explain the possibility of decreased vaginal lubrication while breast-feeding and possible need for use of water-soluble lubricant during intercourse.
   c. Be sure couple understands that fertility will return prior to first menses and that breast-feeding is not adequate contraception.
4. Make provisions for contraception, if desired.
5. Arrange with mother for telephone and clinic follow-up visits.

D. Medical record: document assessment, management plan, and patient teaching

E. Criteria for early discharge of the mother (6-12 hours after delivery)[3]
   1. Mother had normal pregnancy and delivery, i.e., no conduction anesthesia, forceps or vacuum extraction assistance,or excessive blood loss.
   2. Mother has normal postpartum physical and psychosocial status.
   3. All necessary laboratory tests have been drawn or completed for mother; Rh(D) immune globulin (human) has been administered or arrangements have been made for return visit for administration.
   4. Mother can adequately assess her physical condition, care for herself, and recognize postpartum danger signs.
   5. Parents have access to a telephone and transportation should there be a need for consultation or return to a health care facility.
   6. Clinic appointment, office visit, or home visit is scheduled within 72 hours for maternal and infant follow-up.

F. Criteria for early discharge of the infant (6-12 hours)[3]
   1. Baby actively nurses or feeds.
   2. Laboratory tests have been drawn or completed for the baby.
   3. Physical exam is within normal limits, including vital signs, hematocrit, Dextrostix, and indirect Coombs' test.
   4. Birth weight was between 2500 and 4500 g.
   5. Presence of meconium-stained amniotic fluid may preclude discharge.
   6. Gestational age, 37-42 weeks, and size are appropriate to gestational age.
   7. Apgar score is 7 or greater at 1 and 5 minutes.
   8. Parents demonstrate ability to assess infant's physical condition (jaundice, feeding, stooling, voiding, activity level).

V. Interim exam and telephone contacts

A. Purpose of interim contact with family
   1. Provide contact with a health professional during a critical period of transition.
   2. Confirm understanding and compliance with discharge instructions.
   3. Assess infant condition, progress of involution, and perineal healing.

4. Assess psychosocial adjustment and provide appropriate intervention if needed.
5. Provide teaching appropriate to family's situation and identified needs.
6. Promote confidence and independence.

B. Type of contacts
1. Two- or three-day postpartum visit for early-discharge mothers or mothers who have delivered at home[32,42]
2. Two-week postpartum exam
3. Lactation clinic[46]
4. Public health nurse home visit[60]
5. Telephone contact initiated by health care provider[15,26,54]; telephone calls to postpartum mothers are most effective if the caller asks specific open-ended questions (see Appendix A)
6. Parent education or support classes

VI. Six-week postpartum exam (can occur at 4-8 weeks depending on need)

A. Purpose of exam
1. To maintain continuity of care
2. To evaluate physical and emotional condition of mother and screen for abnormalities
3. To provide mother with opportunity to review birth and postpartum experience and discuss any problems with her baby, her family, or herself
4. To observe mother-infant interaction if infant is present
5. To initiate a contraceptive method, if desired

B. Assessment
1. Review chart or available information for the following:
   a. Number of weeks postpartum
   b. Past medical and social history
   c. Details of pregnancy, delivery, and postpartum course
   d. Previous laboratory findings
2. Observe mother for general physical appearance and affect.
3. History: interview mother to complete subjective data base with particular attention to the following:
   a. General health of mother, weight loss or gain since delivery, rest, appetite, fatigue
   b. Problems of pregnancy, delivery, and puerperium
   c. Condition of infant and plans for well-baby care
   d. Family situation and adjustment to newborn
   e. Breast-feeding
   f. Pattern of lochia and return of menses
   g. Present problems
   h. Contraceptive methods used or desired
   i. Resumption of sexual relations and any problems
   j. Emotional status since birth

4. Perform physical examination.
   a. Prepare mother for all procedures and provide for greatest comfort possible.
   b. Take blood pressure, pulse, and weight, if not already done.
   c. Examine breasts for abnormalities of nipples, masses, tenderness, or lactation and teach or review method for self-exam and its importance.
   d. Evaluate heart and lungs.
   e. Palpate abdomen for tenderness, masses, diastasis recti, and involution of uterus.
   f. Examine legs for tenderness, positive Homan's sign, and other indications of thrombophlebitis.
   g. Inspect external genitalia and perineum for lesions and healing of episiotomy or lacerations.
   h. Milk Skene's glands and palpate Bartholin's glands for cysts or abscesses.
   i. Visualize cervix and vaginal walls with speculum and observe for discharge, lesions, inflammation, polyps, eversion, and rugation.
   j. Obtain specimens for Pap smear, gonorrhea culture, *Chlamydia* test, and/or wet mount, when indicated.
   k. Perform bimanual examination to palpate cervix, uterus, and adnexae, determining size, shape, position, abnormalities, and state of involution.
   l. Observe for presence of rectocele or cystocele and integrity of vaginal muscles by having patient contract muscles, bear down, and/or cough.
   m. Perform rectal examination to identify strictures, hemorrhoids, fistulas, or masses.
   n. Fitting of diaphragm, cervical cap, or insertion of IUD may be part of examination if exam is done at 8 weeks or later.
   o. Other portions of physical examination should be included as indicated by history or physical findings.
5. Obtain hematocrit and urine dipstick for glucose and protein and inform mother of the results.

C. Management
1. Order or refer for appropriate treatment for any medical or gynecological problems including any condition whose treatment was deferred until postpartum such as *Trichomonas* vaginal infection or essential hypertension.
2. Interpret findings of exam to woman and explain need for any follow-up or referral, including a 1-year well-woman gynecology examination.
3. Provide appropriate counseling and/or teaching relative to questions initiated by woman or to treatments including the following:
   a. Postpartum exercises: teach Kegel exercises and encourage 50 exercises daily to maintain good perineal muscle tone
   b. Contraception: advantages, disadvantages, and effectiveness of various methods

    c. Diet

    d. Use of medications

    e. Hygiene

    f. Sexuality

    g. Information on working and breast-feeding or how to wean for breast-feeding mothers

  4. Refer mother to appropriate resources, such as the following:

    a. Social services

    b. Public health nurses or visiting nurse association

    c. Well-baby clinics

VII. Postpartum cesarean section examination (2-3 week visit)

A. Purposes of the examination are to:

  1. Maintain continuity of care.

  2. Evaluate physical and emotional condition of mother and screen for abnormalities.

  3. Allow mother to review birth and postpartum experience, particularly her feelings regarding the birth by cesarean section, and to discuss any problems with her baby, family or herself.

  4. Observe mother-infant interaction if infant is present.

  5. Identify a method of contraception, if desired, and initiate if the interval from birth is appropriate for its use.

B. Assessment

  1. Chart review:

    a. Number of weeks postpartum.

    b. Past medical and social history.

    c. Details of pregnancy, delivery, postoperative course.

    d. Previous laboratory findings.

    e. Discharge instructions and medications.

  2. Observe mother for general physical appearance and affect.

  3. History—Interview mother to complete subjective data base with particular attention to:

    a. Wound discharge and/or separation, incisional pain.

    b. Bowel and bladder function.

    c. Lochia pattern, odor, color, amount.

    d. General health of infant and mother.

    e. Family situation and adjustment to newborn.

    f. Feeding problems.

    g. Contraception needs.

    h. Present complaints.

    i. Emotional status since birth.

  4. Perform physical exam.

    a. Prepare mother for all procedures providing for comfort and privacy.

    b. Take blood pressure and pulse.

    c. Examine breasts for masses, tenderness, engorgement, inflammation, abnormal discharge.

    d. Examine surgical scar for induration, redness, drainage, tenderness and approximation.

    e. Gently palpate abdomen for masses, tenderness, hematoma.

  5. Perform other components of physical examination as appropriate.

  6. Collect and interpret laboratory data as indicated by symptomatology, physical findings or history.

C. Management

  1. Consult physician regarding any abnormal findings.

  2. Interpret findings of exam to mother and explain additional procedures and/or referrals as indicated.

  3. Ascertain if mother knows or provide information regarding the type of uterine incision performed and implications for future deliveries.

  4. Provide appropriate counseling and/or teaching in such areas as:

    a. Contraception.

    b. Breast feeding.

    c. General health and hygiene.

    d. Diet.

    e. Resumption of physical activity/exercise.

    f. Medications.

    g. Resumption of sexual activity.

  5. Utilize appropriate referral services such as:

    a. Social/welfare services.

    b. Public Health Nurses/Visiting Nurse Association.

    c. Well-baby clinics.

    d. Cesarean section support groups.

  6. Make arrangements for routine postpartum visit at six weeks.

  7. Document examination findings, management, teaching done and consultations or referrals.

REFERENCES

1. Adams C (ed): Nurse-Midwifery Health Care for Women and Newborns. Orlando, FL, Crune and Stratton, 1983

2. Affonso D: Missing pieces: A study of postpartum feelings. Birth Family Journal 4:159-164, 1977

3. Alternative Birth Center Program Protocols. San Diego, CA, University of California, San Diego Medical Center, 1980

4. Anderson C: Enhancing reciprocity between mother and neonate. Nurs Res 30(2):89-93, 1981

5. Barclay L, Martin N: A sensitive area: Care of the episiotomy in the postpartum period. Aust J Advanced Nurs 1(1):12-19, 1983

6. Bishop B: A guide to assessing parenting capabilities. Am J Nurs 76(11):1784-1787, 1976

7. Braverman J, Roux J: Screening for the patient at risk for postpartum depression. Obstet Gynecol 52(6):731-736, 1978

8. Broussard E: Assessment of the adaptive potential of the mother-infant system: The neonatal perception inventories. Semin Perinatol 3(1):91-100, 1979

9. Buckner E: Use of Brazelton neonatal behavioral assessment in planning care for parents and newborns. JOGN Nurs, 12(1):26-30, 1983

10. Choi E, Hamilton R: The effects of culture on mother-infant interaction. J Obstet Gynecol Neonatal Nurs 15(3):256-261, 1986

11. Curry M: Variables related to adaptation to motherhood in normal primiparious women. J Obstet Gynecol Neonatal Nurs 12(2):115-121, 1983

12. Davidson N: REEDA: Evaluating postpartum healing. J Nurse-Midwifery, 19(2):6-8, 1974

13. Dean P, Morgan P, Towle J: Making baby's acquaintance: A unique attachment strategy. Am J Maternal-Child Nurs 7:37-41, 1982

14. Dodd M: Caring for persons requiring applications of heat and cold, in Sorenson K, Luckmann J (eds): Basic Nursing: A Psychophysiologic Approach. Philadelphia, Saunders, 1979, pp 1145-1172

15. Donaldson N: Fourth trimester follow-up. Am J Nurs 77(7):1176-1178, 1977

16. Droegemueller W: Cold sitz baths for relief of postpartum perineal pain. Clin Obstet Gynecol 23(4):1039-1043, 1983

17. Erickson M: Trends in assessing the newborn and his parents. Am J Maternal Child Nurs (3)2:99-103, 1978

18. Eschenbach D: Acute postpartum infections. Emergency Med Clin North Am 3(1):87-115, 1985

19. Eschenbach D, Rosene K, Tompkins L, et al: Endometrial cultures obtained by a triple-lumen method from afebrile and febrile postpartum women. J Infect Dis 153(6):1038-1045, 1986

20. Ewing T, Smale L, Elliott F: Maternal deaths associated with postpartum vulvar edema. Am J Obstet Gynecol 134(2):173-179, 1979

21. Ezrati J, Gordon H: Puerperal mastitis: Causes, prevention and management. J Nurse-Midwifery, 24(6) 3-8, 1979

22. Filker R, Monif G: The significance of temperature during the first 24 hours postpartum. Obstet Gynecol 53(3):358-361, 1979

23. Funke J, Irby M: An instrument to assess the quality of maternal behavior. JOGN Nurs, 7(5):19-22, 1978

24. Garvey M, Tollefson G: Postpartum depression. J Reprod Med 29(2):113-116, 1984

25. Gordon R: Factors in postpartum emotional adjustment. Obstet Gynecol 25(2):159-166, 1965

26. Haight J: Steadying parents as they go—by phone. Am J Maternal-Child Nursing 2(5)311-312, 1977

27. Halonen J, Passman R: Relaxation training and expectation in the treatment of postpartum distress. J Consult Clin Psychol 53(6):839-845, 1985

28. Harris R: Postpartum urinary tract infection: Role of antimicrobial therapy. Am J Obstet Gynecol 133(2):174-175, 1979

29. Harris R, Thomas V, Hui G: Postpartum surveillance for urinary tract infection: patients at risk of developing pyelonephritis after catheterization. South Med J 70(11):1273-1275, 1977

30. Heffner L, Mennuti M, Rudoff J, et al: Primary management of postpartum vulvovaginal hematomas by angiographic embolization. Am J Perinatol 2(3):204-207, 1985

31. Iffy L, Tenhone W, Grisoli G: Acute myocardial infarction in the puerperium in patients receiving bromocriptine. Am J Obstet Gynecol 155(2):371-372, 1986

32. Jansson P: Early postpartum discharge. Am J Nursing, 85(5):547-550, 1985

33. Jeffcoate T, Miller J, Ross R, et al: Puerperal thromboembolism in relation to the inhibition of lactation by oestrogen therapy. Br Med J 4:19, 1968

34. Katz M, Kroll D, Pak I, et al: Puerperal hypertension, stroke, and seizures after suppression of lactation with bromocriptine. Obstet Gynecol 66(6):822-824, 1985

35. Kennedy J: The high-risk maternal-infant acquaintance process. Nurs Clin North Am 8(3):549-556, 1973

36. Landers D, Green J, Sweet R: Antibiotic use during pregnancy and the postpartum period. Clin Obstet Gynecol 26(2):391-406, 1983

37. Lawrence R: Breast-Feeding: A Guide for the Medical Profession (ed 2). St. Louis, Mosby, 1984

38. Ledger W: The new face of puerperal sepsis. J Obstet Gynecol Neonatal Nurs 3(2):26-32, 1974

39. Ledward R: The management of puerperal hemorrhoids: A double blind clinical trial of Anacal rectal ointment. Practitioner 224:660-661, 1980

40. Ludington-Hoe S: Postpartum: Development of maternicity. Am J Nurs 7(7):1171-1174, 1977

41. Malinowski J: Bladder assessment in the postpartum patient. JOGN Nurs 7(4):14-16, 1978

42. Marecki M: Postpartum follow-up goals and assessment. J Obstet Gynecol Neonatal Nurs 8(4):214-218, 1979

43. Mercer R: The nurse and maternal tasks of early postpartum. Maternal Child Nursing 6:341-345, 1981

44. Meserve Y: Management of postpartum breast engorgement in nonbreastfeeding women by mechanical extraction of milk. J Nurse-Midwifery, 27(3):3-8, 1982

45. Myles M: Textbook for Midwives. Edinburgh: Churchill Livingstone, 1985, p 451

46. Naylor A, Johnson D, Wester R: Teaching health professionals how to promote lactation: Example of a successful program. Unpublished report. San Diego, CA, 1980

47. Nelson G, et al: Timing of postpartum hematocrit determinations. South Med J 73(9):1202-1204, 1980

48. Nichols M: Effective help for the nursing mother. J Obstret Gynecol Neonatal Nursing 7(2):22-30, 1978
49. Noble E: Essential Exercises for the Childbearing Year, (ed 2). Boston, Houghton Mifflin, 1982, pp 58-63
50. Oxorn H: Human Labor and Birth (ed 5). Norwalk, CT, Appleton-Century-Crofts, 1986, pp 865-878
51. Ramler D, Roberts J: A comparison of cold and warm sitz baths for relief of postpartum perineal pain. JOGN Nursing 15(6):471-474, 1986
52. Redlund A: Perineal splinting. Am J Nurs 76(8):1258, 1976
53. Reiser S: A tool to facilitate mother-infant attachment. J Obstret Gynecol Neonatal Nursing 10(4):294-297, 1981
54. Rhode M, Groenjes-Finke J: Evaluation of nurse-initiated telephone calls to postpartum women. Issues Health Care Women 2(2):23-41, 1980
55. Salariya E: Mother-child relationship—FIRST score. J Advanced Nurs 9(6):589-595, 1984
56. Silver D, Harrington M: Thrombophlebitis: Prevention, recognition, and management. Primary Care December, 585-599, 1977
57. Sine I, Cameron J: Relief of afterpains: A deliberative nursing approach. Nurs Clin North Am 3(2):327-336, 1968
58. Sonstegard L, Kowalski K, Jennings B: Women's Health: Volume I. Ambulatory Care. Orlando, FL, Grune & Stratton, 1982
59. Sonstegard L, Kowalski K, Jennings B: Women's Health: Volume II. Childbearing. Orlando, Fl, Grune and Stratton, 1983
60. Stanwick R, Moffat M, Robitaille Y, et al: An evaluation of the routine postnatal public health nurse home visit. Can J Public Health 73:200-205, 1982
61. Sullivan D, Beeman R: Satisfaction with postpartum care: Opportunities for bonding, reconstructing the birth and instruction. Birth Family J 8(3):153-159, 1981
62. Sutton G, Smirz L, Clark D, et al: Group B streptococcal necrotizing fasciitis arising from an episiotomy. Obstet Gynecol 66(5):733-736, 1985
63. Tingle A, Chantler J, Pot K, et al: Postpartum rubella immunization: Association with development of prolonged arthritis, neurological sequelae, and chronic rubella viremia. J Infect Dis 152(3):606-612, 1985
64. Thomsen A, Esperson T, Maigaard S: Cause and treatment of milk stasis, noninfectious inflammation of the breast, and infectious mastitis in nursing women. Am J Obstet Gynecol 149(5):492-495, 1984
65. Thomsen A, Hansen K, Moller B: Leukocyte counts and microbiologic cultivation in the diagnosis of puerperal mastitis. Am J Obstet Gynecol 146(8):938-941, 1983
66. Varney H: Nurse-Midwifery, Boston, Blackwell Scientific, 1980
67. Wadd L: Vietnamese postpartum practices—Implications for nursing in the postpartum period. J Obstet Gynecol Neonatal Nursing 12(4):252-258, 1983
68. Weil A, Reyes H, Rottenberg R, et al: Effect of lumbar epidural analgesia on lower urinary tract function in the immediate postpartum period. Br J Obstet

Gynecol 90:428-432, 1983
69. Whitley N: A Manual of Clinical Obstetrics. Philadelphia, Lippincott, 1985
70. Wong S, Stepp-Gilbert E: Lactation suppression: Nonpharmaceutical versus pharmaceutical methods. J Obstet Gynecol Neonatal Nursing 14(4):302-310.
71. Zepeda M: Selected maternal-infant care practices of Spanish-speaking women. J Obstet Gynecol Neonatal Nursing 11(6):371-374, 1982

APPENDIX A: QUESTIONS FOR POSTPARTUM
TELEPHONE CALLS

1. What questions or problems do you have concerning the care of your baby?

2. How much rest have you been able to get since you have been home?

3. How are you handling visitors?

4. How much help do you have at home?

5. What effect is the new baby in the house having on your family?

6. What questions or problems do you have concerning care of yourself as your body recovers from pregnancy and delivery?

7. What problems have you noticed with the baby blues?

8. Have you thought of any questions about your method of birth control since birth?

Index